Launching Your Dietetics Career

Kyle W. Shadix, MS, RD,
AND *D. Milton Stokes, MPH, RD*
WITH *Jenna A. Bell, PhD, RD*

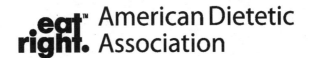

eat™ American Dietetic
right. Association

Diana Faulhaber, Publisher
Laura Pelehach, Acquisitions and Development Manager
Elizabeth Nishiura, Production Manager

10 9 8 7 6 5 4 3 2 1

Library of Congress Cataloging-in-Publication Data

Shadix, Kyle W.
    Launching your dietetics career / Kyle W. Shadix and D. Milton Stokes ; with Jenna A. Bell.
        p. ; cm.
    Includes index.
    ISBN 978-0-88091-439-0
    1. Dietetics—Vocational guidance.   I. Stokes, D. Milton.   II. Bell, Jenna A.
    III. American Dietetic Association.   IV. Title.
    [DNLM: 1. Dietetics. 2. Vocational Guidance. WB 400]
    RM218.5.S53 2011
    613.2023—dc23

2011013618

Contents

About the Authors

Chef Kyle Shadix, MS, RD, CCC, is uniquely qualified in his role as a certified chef de cuisine (CCC), registered dietitian, food scientist, and food safety expert. As a leader in this new terrain that marries cuisine, health, and food science, Chef Kyle wrote for *Today's Dietitian* for almost a decade and now serves on its editorial advisory board. He is a contributing editor for CookingLight.com and a peer reviewer for the journal *Topics in Clinical Nutrition.* He has also written menus for dozens of national consumer and trade magazines, provided menus to various national best-selling nutrition-related books, and contributed to *The World Health and Nutrition Encyclopaedia* (Macmillan Nutrition and Health Reference).

Kyle is an active member of the advisory board for the nutrition department at Teachers College, has served on the Board of the American Institute of Wine and Food, and held numerous key leadership positions with the American Dietetic Association (ADA), the American Culinary Federation, and the International Association of Culinary Professionals. He has received various awards and recognition such as ADA's New York City Recognized Young Dietitian Award, the Emily Quinn Poo Professional Achievement Award from the University of Georgia Alumni Association, and the Publix

Visiting Practitioner at the University of Georgia's Department of Food and Nutrition.

Kyle received his master of science in foods and nutrition from New York University and completed the requirement for becoming an RD at Mount Sinai Medical Center in New York City. He previously graduated with a bachelor of science in consumer foods and food science from the University of Georgia, Athens, and spent his junior year abroad at the Universite d'Orleans, France. He also trained at the Culinary Institute of America, Hyde Park, and Le Cordon Bleu, Paris. Currently Chef Kyle is the corporate senior research chef for PepsiCo Global Beverage R&D, where he strives to reinvent the global portfolio to align with PepsiCo's strategy of making healthier and tastier products. His Web site is www.chefkyle.com.

D. Milton Stokes, MPH, RD, CDN, is a registered dietitian and owner of One Source Nutrition, LLC. He has over 20 years' experience in the areas of food and nutrition as a nutrition professional and former restaurateur.

His firm provides nutrition counseling and consulting to individuals and groups for weight management, eating disorders, and other nutrition-related health conditions. He also partners with companies and organizations to provide nutrition analysis of menus and recipes, recipe testing, presentations on food and nutrition topics, corporate wellness, freelance copy, and more.

In addition, Milton is a former national media spokesperson for the American Dietetic Association; in this capacity he's been featured in *Cooking Light, Fitness, Self, Men's Health,* AOL, *The Washington Post, Ladies' Home Journal,* and countless other media outlets. He's also written freelance articles for *Environmental Nutrition, Today's Dietitian, Family Doctor, Men's Health, Prevention,* WeightWatchers.com, *New York Daily News,* and other publications. His latest book, *Flat Belly Diet! for Men* (Rodale, 2009), is a *New York Times* best seller.

Milton began his RD career in clinical nutrition in New York City, working for a food and nutrition management company. He has served in staff and management positions along the way as well as preceptor for dietetic interns and students from several area colleges and programs. He taught as an adjunct lecturer in the nutrition department at New York University. Milton's graduate degree is in public health from Hunter College, and his clinical training was conducted at Yale-New Haven Hospital. Presently he's earning his PhD in health communication from the University of Connecticut, where he also serves as a teaching assistant and instructor for public speaking, cross-cultural communication, children and media, and an introductory communication course.

Acknowledgments

We gratefully acknowledge the contributions of Jenna A. Bell, PhD, RD, as well as the other individuals who provided profiles, granted interviews, and reviewed drafts for this book. Thanks also to the countless students who have inspired us, the teachers and mentors who started us on our careers, and the hardworking staff at the American Dietetic Association, Commission on Accreditation for Dietetics Education, and Commission on Dietetic Registration.

—*Kyle and Milton*

Introduction

Hi there, reader!

Kyle and Milton here. We want to introduce ourselves since we will be your tour guides through the world of the dietetics student, dietetic intern, and new registered dietitian.

We set out to write this book because we wish we'd had something like this when we were learning the ropes. We have learned a lot that we want to pass along to you so your career journey will be a bit easier.

We plan to help by offering candid advice, solid information, and a good dose of inspiration, courtesy of our esteemed colleagues (see Chapter 7), that will help you stay energized, focused, and productive on your way to becoming a registered dietitian.

Being a registered dietitian is a rewarding career choice, and we hope you love it as much as we do.

Let's go!

— *Kyle and Milton*

1

Welcome to Dietetics!

Congratulations! By opening this book, you've taken a smart shortcut to learning about a career in dietetics—a dynamic and growing profession that is expected to enjoy a 9 percent increase in the 2008–2018 decade, according to the Bureau of Labor Statistics. In 2008, over 60,000 registered dietitians (RDs) worked in hospitals, long-term care facilities, outpatient care centers, physicians' offices, health departments, foodservice agencies, universities, research, schools, federal government, community nutrition, private practice, food industry, media, marketing, supermarkets, and more. With an increasing awareness of just how important food choices are in preventing chronic diseases and improving quality of life, there have never been more diverse opportunities for RDs.

A Spectrum of Career Choices

If you have a passion for food and good health, you may be a great fit for a job in dietetics. Because of the spectrum of jobs in the field, there is no single personality type required for success. As you can see from the list of some of the work environments and job functions for RDs, the profession suits a number of preferences and styles (for more in-depth featured profiles of RDs, see Chapter 7).

Clinical Dietitians

About half of registered dietitians work in a clinical setting, providing nutrition services to patients in hospitals, long-term care facilities, and outpatient clinics. They see patients and assess nutritional needs; provide nutrition diagnoses; develop and implement nutrition plans to address needs; and then monitor, evaluate, and adjust plans along the way as needed. They work with doctors, nurses, speech patholo-gists, and other health care professionals as part of a coordinated health care team. Areas of specialization include cardiovascular

The Future of Practice: A Click Away

With advancements in technology, RDs may increasingly be working with their clients via the Internet, e-mail, and other electronic outlets, so telehealth is a topic to watch. It's an emerg-ing area of practice and we don't have all the answers yet, but here are a few things you should know for now:

- Telehealth is the use of electronic information and telecom-munication technologies to support long-distance clinical health care, patient and professional health-related educa-tion, public health, and health administration.
- There is an opportunity for RDs to be reimbursed for medi-cal nutrition therapy through Medicare Part B. However, to provide telehealth services, you must know the state in which

(continued)

(continued)

> your patients and clients reside, and you must comply with all regulations in that state related to the services you provide. For example, in some states, the first visit must be in person, but follow-ups can be via the phone, Internet, fax, or other forms of electronic communication. Also, if you're based in one state and providing services to another, you may need to be licensed in both states.
>
> - Because telehealth is so new, state licensure boards and the American Dietetic Association (ADA) are still working on resolving a number of questions about it, but the good news is that it's on their radar. You can get up-to-date information by e-mailing the Knowledge Center at knowledge@eatright .org, or you can also peruse some of the FAQs on the topic on the Telehealth page in the members' section of the ADA Web site (www.eatright.org/Members/content.aspx?id=7341).

health, weight management, kidney disease, diabetes, burns, pediatrics, or critical care.

Community Dietitians

Community dietitians work in hunger relief, schools, advocacy organizations, public health clinics, home health agencies, and health maintenance organizations. They may provide nutrition education to individuals and groups about how to eat to prevent disease and promote health. Similarly to clinical dietitians, community dietitians also assess nutritional needs and develop appropriate nutrition care plans. Some community RDs may provide in-home counseling on grocery shopping and food preparation to the elderly, children, and individuals with special needs. Others may advise an organization's nutrition policies or advocacy efforts.

Foodservice Management Dietitians

Foodservice management dietitians are the gatekeepers of food safety, kitchen safety, menu development, budgeting, and planning for small- to large-scale hospitals, companies, and schools. As managers, they may hire, train, and direct other RDs and foodservice workers.

Academic and Research Dietitians

Academic and research dietitians may be involved in clinical lab research, community intervention studies, nutrition education curriculum development, or part of college or university faculty in nutrition programs. There are also faculty opportunities at culinary schools.

Consultant Dietitians

Consultant dietitians have a range of job opportunities. Some work under contract with hospitals or doctors' offices. Some run their own private practices. They conduct nutrition screenings and assessments, and then provide nutrition counseling to improve health. Others work for work-site wellness programs, professional or collegiate sports teams, and supermarkets. Some act as media spokespersons; others are nutrition writers for magazines, books, and other publications.

Industry Dietitians

Jobs in the food industry include roles in public relations; lobbying; research and development in food manufacturing; recipe development and analysis; and commercial writing for brochures and newsletters, advertising, and marketing. Industry dietitians typically work in an office setting.

What, Exactly, *Is* a Registered Dietitian?

The eligibility requirements to be a registered dietitian are established by the Commission on Dietetic Registration (CDR). According to these requirements, becoming an RD means completing academic course work and supervised practice (that is, an internship) and providing verification of completion for both prior to sitting for the RD exam. The academic requirements include a minimum of a baccalaureate degree granted by a U.S. regionally accredited college or university or a foreign equivalent, plus completion of the didactic program in dietetics (DPD) accredited by the Commission on Accreditation for Dietetics Education (CADE), the independent accrediting agency of the ADA.

What Is CDR?

CDR is the credentialing agency for the American Dietetic Association; however, it is an entity separate from ADA. Operating as an 11-member board that includes RDs, dietetic technicians, registered (DTRs), a new RD, and a public representative, CDR protects the public by ensuring that it awards the RD credential and six other credentials to competent candidates.

The supervised practice requirements can be fulfilled through either an accredited dietetic internship program (DI) or an accredited coordinated program in dietetics (CPD). The DI includes at least 1,200 supervised practice hours that takes place after the baccalaureate degree and DPD course work has been completed. The CPD is an academic program in a U.S. regionally accredited college or university that integrates didactic instruction with at least 1,200 hours of supervised practice and culminates in at least a baccalaureate degree.

For a quick profile of the RD, see "At a Glance: Who Is the Registered Dietitian?" (page 6). For more details, keep reading.

The application and process of supervised practice hours will be addressed in Chapter 3, but for now you should note that upon

---

AT A GLANCE: *Who Is the Registered Dietitian?*

A registered dietitian (RD) is someone who:

- Earned at least a bachelor's degree
- Completed the didactic program in dietetics (DPD)
- Fulfilled at least 1,200 hours of supervised practice require-
  ments through a dietetic internship (DI) or coordinated pro-
  gram in dietetics (CPD)
- Passed the Registration Examination for Dietitians
- Maintains their professional development portfolio (PDP)

---

graduation from a CADE-accredited dietetic internship or coordinated program, you may sit for the national registration exam, and a passing score earns you the legally protected title "Registered Dietitian." Some states also offer licensure or certification in the interest of public protection against unqualified practitioners, and it's wise to check with your individual state for details. A listing of state-by-state licensure agencies is available online on the CDR Web site (www.cdrnet.org /certifications).

What Is a Dietetic Technician, Registered?

In this book, we'll focus on what it takes to become an RD, a food and nutrition expert who has received credentials from the Commission on Dietetic Registration. However, you should know that there is another credential given by CDR: the dietetic technician, registered (DTR). These folks work independently or under the supervision of an RD and have their own route to credentialing. That topic deserves the focus of its very own career guide. Similarly to the eligibility requirements to becoming an RD, the path to becoming a DTR includes completing academic course work and supervised practice hours, passing an exam, and maintaining continuing education requirements.

The academic requirements include a minimum of an associate's degree granted by a U.S. regionally accredited college or university or a foreign equivalent, plus completion of a dietetic technician program accredited by CADE, including at least 450 hours of supervised practice. The DTR may work in many of the same settings as the RD, including, but not limited to, hospitals, schools, community nutrition programs, and food companies.

For more information about becoming a DTR, visit the CDR Web site (www.CDRnet.org) as the students' section of the ADA Web site (www.eatright.org/students).

Is an RD Different than a Nutritionist?

Yes! The American Dietetic Association, via its strategic plan, encourages us to adhere uniformly to "RD" and "registered dietitian" to create and reinforce a universal brand identity. It is especially important to differentiate the RD from the "nutritionist" because the RD credential represents competence to provide services to patients and clients, whereas the term "nutritionist" is unregulated. Do a quick Web search for "nutritionist" for an idea of the slew of folks who do not bring the same assurances of education and practice expertise as the RD. However, it is important to note that in reality some RDs call themselves nutritionists, letting their credentials speak for themselves. By working to provide the public with a better understanding of the assurances that accompany the RD credential, ADA hopes its members will be proud to call themselves RDs.

A Closer Look

Nutrition: It's About the Food

By Jonathan Deutsch, PhD

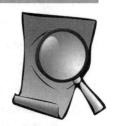

For the past few years I have been teaching foods and cooking classes to nutrition students in DPD programs. That may sound like a fun and easy job. After all, such students are planning to devote their careers to foods—won't they love to learn about food and cooking? For a surprising number of students, the answer is *no*, at least not at first. While nutrition students may be passionate about *aspects* of nutrition and nutrition sciences—encouraging healthful lifestyles in our communities, helping individuals change dietary behavior, or understanding the medical applications of diet—far fewer, it seems, actually want to become RDs because they love to cook and eat and want to encourage others to do the same!

But is it necessary to love food and cooking to be an RD? To illustrate how deeply held our individual and collective relationships with food are, I typically ask my students to write about a food that they would *never* eat and why they would never eat it. You, the reader, might want to try this as well. Class responses range from vegetables and fruits like okra, squash, and durian to meats and meat products like pork, tripe, or chitterlings, to cuisines and preparations like Korean food, sushi, or roasted grasshoppers. Next we discuss *what factors* contribute to the class's strong feelings against these foods. Some answers are:

- "Strange" texture
- Religious prohibitions
- Family memories

- Personal negative experiences
- A "funny feeling"
- Perceived healthfulness
- Cultural preferences
- Taste and personal preferences
- Aroma
- Connection to the living food system
- Perceived food safety
- Unfamiliarity

How do these factors compare to your reasons?

The need for food is not only our primary biological drive, but food is a central and potent channel of communication that carries a rich web of intentions, meanings, and larger forces influencing the way we eat.

Culture, religion, psychology, nutrition, agriculture, economics, marketing, history, and politics all meet around the dinner table to shape how we eat. How we procure, prepare, and serve food is often powerfully negotiated in ways that address larger issues of gender, class, labor, and cultural identities.

Understanding the importance, power, and prominence of food in our lives is the first step to becoming an RD with a healthy understanding of and relationship with food. I encourage aspiring RDs to work through a three-step progression in their relationship with food: love, respect, and understanding.

Understanding is the bare minimum required in an RD's relationship with food. It is the level required by the DPD and by the RD examination. RDs *must* be able to understand the physical and chemical properties of foods themselves; what happens to these properties during cooking, holding, and service; what to look for in purchasing foods; how to prepare foods in a safe and sanitary way; and how to follow procedures such as recipes, formulas, and foodservice systems and how to train others to do so, as well.

Why Understanding? Such an understanding allows RDs to work safely in a hospital or foodservice setting. In a counseling capacity, it allows them to confidently recommend foods and preparations for a client's safe and healthful diet. In food service, it allows them to help chefs and foodservice workers select the best possible ingredients and prepare them in a way that best preserves the flavor, nutritional properties, and texture of the foods.

Respect for food, cooking, and eating makes a good RD better. Having respect for food inspires the RD to pose the *why* question with clients, foodservice workers, and communities to help them better understand and change dietary behavior. Any nutrition student who has taken an introductory foods course knows, for example, that fat plays an important role in "mouth feel," satiety, cooking properties, and flavor. An RD who *understands* this may prescribe a fat reduction for a specific client or setting, whereas one who *respects* these properties will be able to analyze the functions that fat is currently serving while at the same time recommend dietary change in the same circumstance in a way that is more appealing.

Why Respect? In our increasingly diverse world, nutrition wisdom needs to be contextualized for each client and setting. "Eat more fiber" is a less effective recommendation than providing some appealing, easy, cost-effective, flavorful, and culturally specific high-fiber recipes. Understanding not only *what* people are eating but the nutritional, social, cultural, economic, and political *why* helps RDs have a bigger impact. By respecting the food and food habits of an individual or community, RDs can put their nutrition knowledge into action in a way that appeals to clients. Appealing recommendations, programs, and menus are more successful!

Love for food, cooking, and eating make the consummate RD. An RD's passion for a perfectly grilled steak, a vine-ripened tomato eaten whole in the garden, or the pleasure of bok choy steamed with ginger and garlic can inspire a client or class to share in that passion. Such passion can enable positive nutrition advice—instead of simply asking clients to eat *less* in general or less or more of specific nutrients, RDs can encourage people to eat *better* by inspiring them and getting them excited about healthful eating.

Why Love? Loving food allows RDs to innovate not only in programming but in menus and culinary applications of food. An RD who loves food, cooking, and eating can be a holistic food and nutrition professional, by first *understanding* the foods and their properties throughout the cycle; *respecting* these properties and their cultural, social, and personal values; and *loving* the foods, the pleasures of the table, and the sensual properties of food shopping, cooking, eating, and serving. In the same way that a passionate teacher can inspire a love of learning in her or his students, an RD passionate about food can inspire a healthful, respectful, and safe relationship with food in her or his clients and communities.

Jonathan Deutsch is assistant professor and director of Foods Program, Department of Tourism and Hospitality, Kingsborough Community College, City University of New York.

2

Hitting the Books

Once you've made the choice to follow your passion for nutrition, you'll want to choose an academic program that's right for you. This chapter will provide resources for researching programs and provide an overview of what to expect from the academic portion of your path to the registered dietitian (RD) credential, including the course work (that is, the didactic program in dietetics [DPD]), various degrees you may pursue, and suggested extracurricular activities.

Essentially, before sitting for the exam to become an RD, you will need to complete an academic program from an accredited school then put in a considerable number of hours "on the job," typically in the form of an internship (for more information on internships, see Chapter 3). This chapter focuses on the required schooling and addresses undergraduates, graduate students, and career changers.

Finding Your Best Program

To find a program that is a good fit, start by being honest about what you want to get out of your experience. For example, you may ask yourself how well a program will prepare you for a career in the area of practice of your choice, be it clinical, private practice, community, or research, to name just a few. Perhaps you also have practical things to consider, like geography, tuition costs, or preference for an urban, suburban, or rural setting.

The geographic location of where you study is an important consideration on more than a personal level; on a professional level, it will influence the kinds of work and volunteer opportunities available to you (for example, a semester working on an organic farm versus leading nutrition education classes for public schools in an major city).

You'll also want to do your homework and speak to current students and faculty as well as former students to get firsthand insights into a program. It's a good idea to speak to a range of students, including those who may have similar goals for the future or who have a similar educational background (this may be especially useful for the career changer). In the end, only you can decide if a program is right for you, and doing the legwork will make the choice easier. Find additional tips in "Researching Programs: The Basics" (page 17). The bottom line is that you want to find the program that will match your interests, build on your strengths, and bolster your weaknesses.

Overview of Dietetics Education

The Commission on Accreditation for Dietetics Education (CADE; pronounced KAY-dee) of the American Dietetic Association (ADA) is the independent accrediting agency for dietetics education. To become an RD, you must complete your education through a CADE-accredited program, which ensures that you've met its standards for knowledge requirements and competencies for an entry-level dietitian. The current standards (from 2008) are available on the CADE Web site in the Curriculums section (www.eatright.org/CADE /content.aspx?id=149).

The two main paths for completing the educational requirements are:

- The **didactic program in dietetics** (DPD), followed by an internship (supervised practice)
- The **coordinated program in dietetics** (CPD), which includes supervised practice (an internship)

Didactic Program in Dietetics Followed by an Internship

The DPD refers specifically to the academic classes you need to complete before applying for a dietetic internship. When CADE accredits a program, it verifies that the program covers specific knowledge areas in food, nutrition, foodservice management, clinical care, community care, health care systems, and other areas. Course titles may vary from one university to another, even in the same state, but ultimately, students in a CADE-accredited DPD will be satisfying the required knowledge areas (see "Sample DPD Course Listings" on page 16). There are currently (as of 2011) 226 accredited DPDs, most of which are targeted to undergraduate students; 8 of these programs result in a graduate degree. See the box titled "Researching Programs: The Basics" (page 17) for suggestions on how to investigate your DPD options.

Did You Know?

The word "didactic" comes from the Greek *didaktikos,* which means literally "to teach."

Sample DPD Course Listings

Sample DPD Courses at University A		Sample DPD Courses at University B	
Course	**Credits**	**Course**	**Credits**
Biostatistics	3	Introduction to Modern Chemistry	5
Chemistry of Food	3		
Food Policy and Food Safety	3	Principles of Organic Chemistry	5
Food Policy and Food Safety Lab	2	Food Microbiology and Sanitation	3
Protein and Carbohydrate	4	Nutritional Biochemistry	3
Lipid Metabolism	4	Principles of Human Anatomy and Physiology	3
Vitamin and Mineral Nutrition	4	Nutrition and Health	3
Evaluation of Nutrition Status	3	Diet Assessment and Planning	3
Community Nutrition	3	Nutrition and the Life Cycle	3
Nutrition Education Principles and Practice	3	Clinical Nutrition Assessment and Intervention	3
Nutrition and Chronic Disease	4	Community Nutrition	3
Medical Nutrition Therapy I	2	Introduction to Foods and Food Science	3
Nutrition in Acute Care	4	Food Management Theory	3
Medical Nutrition Therapy II	2	Food Production and Management	3
Management of Nutrition Services	4	Food Science and Technology	3

Coordinated Program in Dietetics

A coordinated program in dietetics synchronizes both the dietetics class work and the required 1,200 hours of supervised practice/internship. CPDs are ideal for students who know before they start college or graduate school that they want to become an RD. In 2011, there were 53 accredited CPDs; 21 of them resulted in a graduate degree.

The **undergraduate student** usually applies for a CPD during the sophomore year, and the junior and senior year include the supervised practice (the dietetic internship).

Researching Programs: The Basics

- The American Dietetic Association offers useful information about CADE-accredited DPDs and CPDs across the country on the CADE Web site (www.eatright.org/CADE-DPD and www.eatright.org/CADE-CP). You can use this online resource to sort programs by state, programs offering distance education or course credit transfer agreements, and those that result in a graduate degree.
- Visit programs' Web sites to learn more. Look for:
  - A **physical address**, which gives you an idea of the geography and environment.
  - **Department name**, which provides an idea about a program's focus and strengths (for example, nutrition and food science, health policy, wellness, family and consumer sciences, hospitality management, human environmental sciences, nursing or medical schools, nutrition and exercise, and more).
  - The name and contact information of **the program director** so that you can get in touch via phone, fax, or e-mail.
  - Important **basic facts,** such as annual enrollment size and timing, tuition, degrees granted, and alternative education options (such as evening or independent study).

The **graduate student** usually applies to a graduate program that includes a CPD. Some graduate schools will transfer certain course credits from undergraduate institutions; plus, some graduate courses will qualify toward both the graduate degree and CPD core competencies. It is best to work with an individual program's CPD director for personalized academic planning.

To find out more about CDP programs, see the box titled "Researching Programs: The Basics" (page 17).

The Career Change: Advanced Degree Programs

A graduate program is an option for career changers with undergraduate degrees in areas other than dietetics. As noted in previous sections, both DPDs and CPDs that result in graduate degrees are available. In 2011, there were 21 CPDs and 8 DPDs that could result in a graduate degree.

If you're coming from a nonscience field, you may have questions about the science requirements. Science is part of the foundation of nutrition, from organic chemistry, in which you'll examine the structure of glucose, to food science, in which you can expect to study the Maillard reaction that occurs when food browns in the cooking process. If dietetics is your field, you should be prepared for a heavy load of the physical sciences, which can be challenging but is fundamental to building a good understanding of nutrition and human health. Expect to take science courses that cover the following topics: general chemistry, inorganic chemistry, organic chemistry, biochemistry, anatomy, physiology, general biology, microbiology, and food science. A positive attitude, good classroom and study skills, access to a tutor or study groups, and a commitment to succeed will all help you make it through what many students consider the most challenging classes in their academic careers, whether they are undergraduates, graduate students, or career changers.

Tips for Career Changers

- **Working while going to school?** Consider looking into tuition reimbursement from your current job. As a part-time student, you may want to limit your course load to one to two courses per semester, as each hour of class time may require one to three hours of work outside of class.
- **Coming from a nonscience background?** Be encouraged by the fact that many of today's RDs who started in another field have successfully excelled in the sciences. Ask your program director to put you in touch with former students who made the switch and get their take on how to navigate the challenges.

Your Degree Options

BS, BA, MS, MA, MPH, MBA, PhD, DrPh, EdD, ScD, DCN—in dietetics and nutrition, we're big on listing our degrees and credentials. They show others, especially patients and clients, that we've earned the right to care for them and provide services. If a big-name client, such as a public relations firm in New York City, wants RDs for a focus group, it will recruit RDs, not anyone else. Another employer may specify that a successful applicant possess a graduate degree in a particular area, such as foodservice management, clinical dietetics, or nutrition communication. So let's take a tour of the alphabet city of degrees and look at each one.

A Closer Look

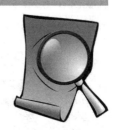

Highlighting a Unique Program
for the 21st Century:
The Culinary Nutrition Program
at Johnson & Wales University

Johnson & Wales was the first to offer bachelor's degrees in culinary arts and baking and pastry arts. Now another first: a bachelor of science in culinary nutrition—a hands-on culinary nutrition degree, the first in the country accredited by CADE. This program is designed for students who seek to apply nutrition principles and scientific knowledge to their culinary arts skills. Courses are taught by professional chefs and registered dietitians.

The goal of the culinary nutrition degree program is to impart the technical and cognitive skills required of a self-reliant professional who can:

- Manage the delivery of quality nutrition services to diverse populations.
- Incorporate current nutrition theory into classic cuisine.
- Assure that foodservice operations meet the food and nutrition needs of clients.
- Supervise the daily operations of a foodservice facility.
- Participate in activities that promote nutrition and the profession of dietetics.

Bachelor's Degrees

Undergraduate programs grant bachelor's degrees. Those are signified most often as either BS or BA; the former for bachelor of science, and the latter for bachelor of arts. Many RDs complete their DPD during their undergraduate career before entering a dietetic internship (DI).

Master's Degrees in Nutrition

Master's degrees are for those who want to pursue advanced study and training for specialized positions or roles in management, administration, and research. For example, a position as director of food and nutrition at a hospital or food company may require master's preparation.

Master's degree candidates may already be RDs, having completed a DPD and DI in their undergraduate days. They may also be career changers who have their bachelor's degree in a non-nutrition area and are simultaneously working toward completing a DPD, DI, and graduate degree.

Students can expect to take approximately 30 to 45 (or more) credits toward nutrition, psychology, public health, research methods, epidemiology, communication, or health care administration to earn a master of science (MS) or master of arts (MA) degree. Of course, there are many more areas to study; we only listed a few to illustrate our point. There is also usually a thesis, comprehensive exam, or culminating project for any master's level degree.

You may have also seen the MSEd or MEd credential, which are master's level degrees in education, such as health education or nutrition education. One example is the Columbia University Teachers College program in community nutrition education, which requires 60 credits. Graduates with a master's degree in nutrition education are qualified for a number of roles, including curriculum development, policy advisement, health care, research, and academia.

Complementary Master's Degrees

In addition to the MS, MA, MSEd, or MEd in nutrition, dietetics students may also be interested in degrees in public health (master of public health, or MPH) or business (master of business administration, or MBA). These tend to require from 40 to 60 credits, or more, depending upon the school's curriculum. An MPH prepares a student to work in community health and nutrition, research, administration, and public policy development, while an MBA helps graduates cultivate expertise in business, management, economics, and human resources, among other areas.

Doctoral Degrees

Your professors likely have doctoral degrees. A PhD, or doctorate in philosophy, is one of the more popular degrees, but there are others, such as doctorate in public health (DrPH), doctorate in science (ScD), and doctorate in education (EdD). These programs usually require 70 credits or more, a research project, dissertation, and successful completion of comprehensive exams. For individuals seeking advanced clinical training and skills, the University of Medicine and Dentistry of New Jersey developed a doctor of clinical nutrition (DCN) degree in 2003. These students complete a clinical doctoral residency as well as a research project.

Out of the Classroom and into the Real World (Kind of)

As a dietetics student, fieldwork, independent study, volunteering, and summer internships are all great ways to jump out of the classroom and into the real world. You may even be able to receive academic credit for your time.

There's no doubt about it: seeking educational experiences outside the classroom is good for you. You'll gain real world experience and perhaps learn a thing or two about your professional likes and, just as importantly, your dislikes. Plus, you have the opportunity to make valuable contacts who may provide you with great recommendation letters and may even become nurturing mentors.

Before you embark on any of these experiences, evaluate your current status as a student. How much time can you reasonably commit to non-classroom activities? In what type of environment do you thrive—a bustling public health clinic or a quiet medical laboratory? Can you work with demanding people? Are your grades up to par? How far are you willing to travel? Answering these questions and more will help you narrow your options.

Fieldwork and Independent Study

In addition to excelling as a student, you can enrich your educational experience through nutrition-related fieldwork or independent study that is meant to be done concurrently and in complement to your academic work. Your professors and academic advisers are great resources to find out about relevant opportunities in the community.

Some academic programs include mandatory fieldwork for credit (for example, volunteering at a local soup kitchen during a community nutrition course). However, whether it is required or not, you will benefit from fieldwork because it lets you take what you learned in the classroom and apply that knowledge in the real world. Showing some work experience in the field may also give you an edge when it comes time to apply for dietetic internship programs (see Chapter 3). You may seek experiences that focus on wellness, public health, foodservice management, nutrition in ambulatory care, home health care, and clinical services. Your program director can arrange your fieldwork for you or at least point you in the right direction. If you're responsible for arranging your own fieldwork, you can find helpful strategies in the section later in this chapter about securing a summer internship.

The primary purpose of fieldwork is to provide the opportunity to integrate academic knowledge with the application of skills at progressively higher levels of performance and responsibility. The "real world" setting emphasizes the direct application of this knowledge through supervised intervention with the public. Fieldwork permits students the opportunity to gain real-life work experience that increases their skills, knowledge of the dietetics field, and useful contacts for future employment. Field work is also an opportunity to carry out projects that contribute to your overall growth and an occasion to develop a network and seek a mentor.

Independent study is a structured way to gain experience that goes above and beyond your didactic program, allowing you the chance to explore academic materials or topics that are unavailable or not fully developed in standard courses. For example, you could arrange with an instructor to independently study an area of dietetics that interests you (such as eating disorders, restaurant management, or the practice of dietetics in overseas populations) through a reading project or a combination of book work and laboratory work. Gaining this experience (and showing the initiative to go after it) certainly doesn't hurt when it comes time to apply for the dietetic internship; plus, some schools will provide credit for this work. To get academic credit, you will need to find a faculty member at your school to supervise your independent study class. Check with your program director for specific advice.

Volunteering

There is an unwritten rule in dietetics: you *must* volunteer! Ideally you should try to volunteer with a cause that is food-related, and if possible, nutrition-specific. Hospitals are an ideal place to gain that experience, but you cannot always be guaranteed a spot with the RDs. Many prospective dietetic interns end up working at an intensive care unit's information desk or for community affairs or public relations offices. Do not worry if you don't end up working directly with an RD. What counts is that you gave your valuable time to a worthy cause, and this evidence is invaluable on your future applications. Of course, a letter of recommendation from the volunteer coordinator won't hurt, either.

Volunteering shows you have an interest in the community, and it's a way to practice your talents and learn new skills. For example, if you give your time to the local hospital to help the RDs organize and create educational materials, that may lead to health fair opportunities where you can practice teaching others what nutrition knowledge you have gained so far. If your knowledge is limited because you have only taken one or two classes, you can observe the pros while they chat up folks at the health fair. Shadowing and listening to registered dietitians early on makes an impact on your education and your future career path.

Volunteering also helps to make you well-rounded. You'll learn skills that are transferable to other settings—the classroom, internship, and jobs—and you'll demonstrate that you have what it takes to plan ahead and manage your time, as well as your

Student Volunteers Make a Difference

The Greater New York Dietetic Association is partially run by students. Surprised? Each time the association has an official function, students participate in discussions and contribute ideas and suggestions for operational issues. They assist with set up and clean up for conferences and meetings, staff registration tables at seminars, and do so much more. Wherever there is a committee chair or executive officer, you can bet students are close by, and you can bet they were there all along, taking part in planning the meetings and seeing the events and meetings through to successful completion. The wonderful students in New York City should inspire you to try and do the same. Never say, "I want to help, but I'm only a student." Students *can* run the show!

willingness to serve others. If you can attend college, work part time, and volunteer 8 to 10 hours per week, this proves you are balanced.

If you feel unsure where to start with volunteering, make an appointment with your adviser or program director. You can even talk with one of your professors. He or she may have community connections, which may be useful if you didn't grow up in the area where you are now attending school. Consider working within health departments, nutrition education programs, hunger relief organizations such as a food bank, WIC (Special Supplemental Nutrition Program for Women, Infants, and Children) centers, farmer's market educational programs, or family resource centers. Call them up. They may accept volunteers, or they may refer you to another agency in greater need.

Summer Internships

Not to be confused with the structured dietetic internship that is required before sitting for the RD exam, a summer internship is an optional opportunity to gain additional work experience in areas of interest.

What are the benefits? You may be thinking about how busy you are all semester long taking notes and studying for exams (and perhaps volunteering in your local soup kitchen once a week!). You may want to spend your summer relaxing, going on vacation to some exotic destination, or venturing out for gainful employment. After all, you need to rest and make a little cash for the future. Well, believe us, a summer internship *is* investing in your future. Plus, it's a little different from volunteering during the school year because you have the chance to spend more time immersed in a project.

Don't know where you want to work? The same rules apply here as they do for finding great fieldwork, independent study, and volunteer opportunities: start by tapping the resources available to you. First, check what's accessible on campus. Is there a medical center, student health service, outpatient clinic, or counseling and testing center where you can work or volunteer to gain experience? What about opportunities in the community surrounding your school or neighboring cities? Look for hospitals, long-term care facilities (such as nursing homes and assisted-living facilities), hospices, and adult and pediatric day care facilities. Also check with local health departments. They may hire you for paid or volunteer experience working with WIC clients, Food Stamp recipients, a diabetes children's camp, or individuals who plan and receive food from Meals on Wheels.

Once you have your eye on specific programs:

- Contact them directly.
- Call and ask to speak with a manager or a director to find out if they are hiring or taking on volunteers. Many facilities and organizations are eager to accept students.
- Consult with your program adviser to help determine a list of goals to accomplish during your experience.
- Send out resumes with letters of introduction describing who you are, your special skills, and what you hope to contribute and learn from the experience.

Selected Organizations that Look for Volunteers

- United Way
- American Cancer Society
- Red Cross
- Local health departments
- Food banks
- VolunteerMatch.org
- 1-800-Volunteer.org

Mentors

It's never too early in your dietetics career to be on the lookout for a great mentor. Whether you're studying dietetics as an undergraduate or as someone with 20 years' experience in a different profession, having someone you can look to for guidance, counseling, and advice about the nutrition world is valuable.

This person has been there and done that. You can bet she or he was in your shoes at one point, made all the mistakes, learned from them, and moved on to other exciting challenges. That doesn't mean, however, a mentor always has the answers and directs your every move. You want to make your own way—but it helps to bounce ideas off of someone you trust. Balancing your decisions with the wisdom of experienced practitioners will serve you well. Guidance from a mentor can help set you apart as you venture down your career path, even in the educational stages.

So, where do you find a mentor? Educators are mentors. Get to know yours well, especially those in your department. Spend time with your adviser and/or major professor. Develop a relationship so you know your teachers and they know you. These people have your future in their hands when it comes time to write recommendation letters for internship appointments, scholarships, and employment. However, school isn't the only place to find a mentor.

Survey your surroundings and look for someone you admire and respect. Do you know a community member, local business person, church leader, relative, or educator in another department, school, or program?

It's a good idea to spend time with potential mentors and develop a relationship. Once the two of you are comfortable, ask the person if he or she will consider serving as your mentor. Some people may feel honored, while others are surprised. Explain what you can offer and what you hope to gain in a mentor-mentee partnership. That way your expectations are clear.

Once you have been matched with a dietetic internship, you will be eligible to join ADA as a student member, and you can and should take advantage of all of the dietetic practice groups and networking groups that have mentor programs.

A Closer Look

Mentors Pave the Way to Success

By Martha Rosenau, RD.

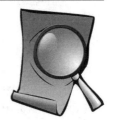

In the last year I have served as a mentor to students, interns, and dietitians preparing to go into private practice. As a mentor, I provide guidance and encouragement, suggest resources, provide ideas, and share my own experiences. As someone who just began a private practice not that long ago, I believe I can offer a fresh perspective on how to navigate the start-up phase.

Those that I mentor frequently express concerns and uncertainty with starting their own business. They need reassurance that their business model is sound and that they will be able to support themselves financially. It is not surprising that these fears surface during mentoring sessions. Taking the leap into the unknown and letting go of a paycheck is a universally terrifying experience. In these types of conversations, I always encourage my mentees to follow their dreams. I try to help them work through their fears, so that they can keep moving forward. Often by just listening to someone's concerns, I have done more for them than by providing sage advice or guidance.

What I have learned from mentoring is that there is no one-size-fits all or *right* way of starting a private practice. The best advice I can give to mentees is to have a well-developed business plan. After all, by researching the competition, having a dynamic marketing plan, and evaluating all sources of potential income, they are more likely to succeed. Usually mentees contact me before they have written their business plan. In these instances, I encourage them to contact a Small Business Development Center or SCORE to get help with this key aspect of starting a new business (for more information, visit the U.S. Small Business Administration Web site: www .sba.gov).

In reviewing mentees' strengths, I find that most come to private practice with significant clinical skills but little experience in accounting and marketing. By understanding what their strengths and weaknesses are, I can steer them toward resources and educational opportunities that would benefit them the most. If I am asked about an area of private practice that I do not have experience in (such as taking insurance), I refer them to another dietitian in this field who can better serve their needs.

Mentoring has been deeply rewarding for me. The greatest gifts I have received from mentoring are thank-you notes from students and dietitians. I prominently display these cards in my office to remind me that there is more to running a business than dollars and cents. Another unexpected benefit is the renewed enthusiasm I have for my work. Mentoring is a two-way exchange of thoughts and inspiration that frequently gives me new ideas to incorporate in my marketing plan. No matter how many dietitians I mentor, I continue to find the experience profoundly satisfying and I look forward to each new match.

Adapted with permission from Ventures *(Nutrition Entrepreneurs DPG newsletter). Spring 2008; p. 4.*

3

The Nitty-Gritty Details of the Dietetic Internship

A major milestone in your journey to becoming a registered dietitian (RD) is the dietetic internship. It's also known as the "DI" or just "the internship" and comes after you've fulfilled the didactic program in dietetics (DPD) requirements, but before you're allowed to sit for the RD exam.

The reality is that being accepted into a DI is a competitive process, and there is concern about the ratio of applicants to available spots. For example, in April 2010, 2,076 of 4,169 applicants were matched to a DI. The April 2009 match was similar, with a large number of applicants and a match rate of 50 percent. In addition to shortage concerns, the process of researching and applying for an internship can be intimidating in and of itself.

We're here to help. This chapter will provide an overview of the DI, breaking it down into its components. Then we'll provide suggestions for finding the right kind of DI for you, as well as a couple of great interviews that offer advice to applicants. We'll go over the details of putting together a winning application and offer interviewing tips for the internships that include an interview in the application process. Financial aid considerations are covered at the end of the chapter.

Dietetic Internships 101

The dietetic internship is designed to prepare students to meet the performance requirements for entry-level RDs. As of 2010, an internship must provide at least 1,200 hours of supervised practice. Internships may span anywhere from 6 to 24 months, with most falling in the 10- to 12-month range.

Your supervised practice takes place in health care, community, and management settings under the guidance of a preceptor (an RD or other professional who has the appropriate knowledge, experience, and credentialing/licensure [if applicable] in the area in which he or she is supervising interns, as determined by your internship director). In 2011 there were 243 CADE-accredited dietetic internships, 37 of which offered a graduate degree.

> ### Word on the Web
>
> Learn from people who understand the challenges of being a dietetic intern! **All Access Internships** (www .AllAccessInternships.com) has a running list of dietetics student and DI bloggers in the Links page of the Resources section.
>
> All Access Internships also provides Webinars, help with the application process, and a wealth of other information for prospective interns.

As mentioned in Chapter 2, before you can apply for a dietetic internship, you must complete at least a bachelor's degree and the DPD course requirements. You must also supply either the *declaration of intent to complete form* or a *verification statement form*. If your undergraduate degree is not connected to your DPD studies, the DI will also need an official copy of your transcripts from the registrar of the college or university you attended, to verify you have completed a bachelor's degree.

Your didactic program director is responsible for completing these forms for you and should work with you when the time comes. Only the program director of your CADE-accredited dietetics education program can sign your declaration of intent to complete form

Researching the Dietetic Internship: The Basics

The American Dietetic Association offers useful information about CADE-accredited dietetic internships across the country on the CADE Web site (www.eatright.org/CADE-DI), including:

- The ability to sort programs by state, by programs offering distance education, and by programs that may result in a graduate degree.
- Links to Web sites that you can visit to learn more about a program.
- A physical address for each program, which gives you an idea of the geography and environment.
- Each program's department name and area of concentration, which tells you a program's DI focus (such as public health, management, nutrition therapy, research, education, sports nutrition, and more).
- The name and contact information of the program director so that you can get in touch via phone, fax, or e-mail.
- Important basic facts, such as annual enrollment size and timing; length of program (typically from 6 to 24 months); tuition; degrees granted; stipends, if available; and timing for the matching process, so you know when to apply.

and verification statement form. If you are applying to a DI while you are still in school, she or he will review your transcripts, complete and sign the declaration of intent to complete form for you to include in your dietetic internship application. When you are ready to graduate from your college or university, your program director will evaluate your transcript to make sure all DPD requirements have been met, check with your school's registrar to confirm that you have been approved for graduation (no outstanding bills, fines, or other issues), and issue you at least six copies of your verification statement. Do not lose these! You must give one copy to your DI, and you may need others for your state licensing board, graduate school, or employer.

Most DIs use a computer matching system to match applicants to internships (more on this a little later in the chapter), and you can contact individual programs for their application deadlines.

Anatomy of an Internship

A dietetic internship has three parts: clinical care (also known as nutrition therapy or medical nutrition therapy [MNT]), food systems management, and community nutrition. In each part, your internship may be further segmented into rotations. All internships offer staff relief, and some may offer an elective option.

Clinical Care/Medical Nutrition Therapy

The MNT experience includes several rotations designed to give you broad-based, in-depth experiences in clinical care. In addition to a general nutrition therapy rotation, you may rotate through specialty areas, such as research, renal, diabetes, nutrition support/critical care, rehabilitation, geriatric, psychiatry, pediatrics, and transplant. As you progress in the program, you will be given more responsibility and increased patient assignments and learning experiences. Toward the end of your clinical rotations, you will be expected to assume the full

Special Interest or Elective Rotations

Although internships are designed with a specific concentration (see "Researching the Dietetic Internship: The Basics" on page 33), some offer students the opportunity to coordinate their own special rotations, or electives. Special interest rotations can last from one week to six weeks, and the experience all depends on the intern. This is the time to go for something you haven't yet learned in the internship or a chance to build on your past experiences in an area of practice you know you're interested in.

Suggestions and ideas for special interest rotations:

- Medical nutrition product sales
- Research (lab and clinical trials)
- Food manufacturing
- Food and nutrition organizations (for example, the International Food Information Council or American Dietetic Association)
- Health or nutrition media
- Burn clinic
- Pediatric hospital
- Nursing home
- Private practice dietitian
- Chef and culinary staff in home-meal delivery program
- Bariatric surgery clinic
- Radiation and chemotherapy practice
- Hemodialysis unit
- Foodservice distributor
- Restaurant/sanitation inspector

responsibilities of a dietitian and function like the RD for an assigned area (length of time in this role varies by program, which is sometimes referred to as "staff relief").

Overall, the staff relief experiences help you to see what it will be like to work as an RD on your own. The experiences help foster self-confidence in basic skills as well as professionalism in the field. Of course, you'll have access to other RDs/preceptors who can assist you if the need arises, but this is an opportunity to demonstrate that you are capable of running your own show, so to speak.

Food Systems Management

The food systems management experience lets you practice in a variety of foodservice and management situations. Rotations may include the food production and service area, management, and administration. You will apply your knowledge of food systems management to learning how RDs function in the management and administrative area of dietetics. Some programs may focus on management experience and do not include a foodservice portion.

In this part of your internship, you may work with the food purchasing manager (also called "procurement"), frontline supervisors who manage the tray-line staff, the executive chef and/or production manager who coordinates food preparation, as well as other professionals.

Community

In the community nutrition rotation, you apply the principles of nutrition to various groups of people in the community environment. Rotations may include experiences with various community programs and community agencies, and you may have the opportunity to work in diverse settings. Options include your local health department, food banks, cooperative extensions, school nutrition programs, senior nutrition programs, WIC (Special Supplemental Nutrition Program for Women, Infants, and Children), Head Start, United Way, and more.

You might counsel clients to encourage good nutrition and eating habits as well as teach classes on a variety of topics, such as prenatal nutrition, healthful eating on a budget, and tips for feeding toddlers. You might also find yourself evaluating grants, creating nutrition education materials, or leading supermarket tours of healthful foods.

Make the Most of Every Rotation

Now that we've provided an overview of the kinds of activities you might encounter throughout your internship, we'd like to emphasize that it is just that—an overview. Internships vary, and so will the organizations and projects you work with. It's a smart idea to ask for advice about the possible projects, goals, and objectives you can set for yourself in each rotation. You should plan to tap your program director and each individual preceptor for their guidance in this area.

Distance Education and Internet Education

Distance programs originated to provide experiences in geographic areas where no formal dietetic internship or coordinated program was available. These programs may be right for you if your family or job responsibilities keep you in an area that may not have a DI or coordinated program in dietetics (CPD). In 2011, 12 programs offered distance education.

Distance education programs often include an initial one-week, on-campus orientation program, after which instruction, courses, assignments, and advisement are given via the Internet or phone. Arrangements for transportation, meals, and lodging for the on-campus orientation are usually the responsibility of the intern.

For More Information

You can find a current list of distance education programs with contact information on the CADE Web site (www.eatright .org/CADE-DI).

In general, the distance education intern will need to coordinate much more of his or her own internship experience and may find it challenging to find sites and preceptors. Your preceptors and facilities will be subject to approval by the dietetic internship director, and facilities providing supervised practice must sign a contract. A benefit is that you will be networking with colleagues and organizations in your own area.

To learn whether a distance education internship is a good option for you, contact the programs that offer distance education and ask to speak with the program director, as well as current and former interns. Ask about the logistics of how the internship works, its challenges, and any strategies to overcome those challenges.

A Closer Look

Finding the Right Internship for You

This section provides insights from a recent intern's perspective. Kyle and Milton interview Jenny Westercamp, RD, chief executive officer, All Access Internships; sports nutrition consultant at SportFuel, Inc.; and author of Getting Matched: A Guide for Dietetics Students *(available from www.AllAccessInternships.com).*

Kyle and Milton: As a relatively recent dietetic intern yourself and cofounder of AllAccessInternships.com, a peer-to-peer resource for aspiring RDs, what is the most important thing an applicant needs to know about the DI?

Jenny: The dietetic internship is the transition between student and professional. Looking at the bright side of an additional year of training, we are lucky to have this time to evolve without having to dive right into a 9 to 5 job. With that being said, the responsibilities of both a student and a professional are still given to you. You will have projects and homework assignments on top of clocking in from at least 9 to 5 (for most full-time programs, anyways). Balance will be a running theme throughout the internship—balancing work, assignments, and fun, too! Overall, it is definitely an experience that will help you grow both personally and professionally and prepare you well for the real world.

K & M: What's your advice on what to consider when looking for a good match?

Jenny: Many factors differentiate each internship program from the other. These include location, expense, emphasis, length, rotation locations, elective rotation options, graduate credit options, or distance internship options, to name a few. Consider what you can realistically afford to do and choose from programs that will match your interests and experiences. I was willing to look across the country for internships. I knew I wanted a general emphasis, was attracted to teaching hospitals, did not want a graduate degree, and wanted the option to do an elective rotation in my hometown no matter where my internship was located. Massachusetts General Hospital provided all of that, and that is where I got matched. When you apply to programs that match what you are interested in, your genuine enthusiasm for the program will shine through to the selection committee and will reflect well on your application. The "match" works two ways—both you and the program should fit well with each other. Proving you are the perfect fit is what the application is for!

K & M: What's the best way for the DI applicant to evaluate a program?

Jenny: Learn about the rotations and the level of responsibility you will have at these rotation sites. Are rotation sites accustomed to having interns? Will you be mostly observing or mostly participating in tasks? Talk with former interns about their experiences (both the pros and the cons of the program). Decide if the "internship culture" is attractive to you (that is, the director's work style, department culture, and institution culture).

K & M: Is there a magic number for how many they should apply to?

Jenny: If you apply to programs with preselection, without ranking and computer matching, then apply to as many of those as you would like (just like college admissions). Your chances of applying are the same with each program. When applying to programs with computer matching, though, your chances of acceptance by these programs will vary based on your rankings. It is impossible to predict the effect that ranking a program 1 or 6 will have on your chances, as this is dependent on how many people apply to those programs and also rank the programs high. In general, four to five programs is a good recommendation.

K & M: Are there networking groups you recommend where applicants can learn about others' experiences?

Jenny: All Access Internships has an always-expanding collection of testimonials from former interns on their experiences—this is our users' favorite feature. There is also contact information for past interns listed so that students can contact them directly. Ask the dietetic internship directors or your didactic program director for intern contact information, too. In addition, the American Dietetic Association Student Community of Interest (http://eatright .communityzero.com/students) is a good resource, as well as your state's student dietetic association.

K & M: Anything else you wish to add?

Jenny: My best advice for surviving the application process and the internship is summed up in this quote by John Wooden: "Things turn out best for the people who make the best of the way things turn out." No matter what happens on the road to the RD (the stress of the application process and the challenges that come before you in the internship), having a positive attitude every step of the way will be one of the most important keys to your success as a student, intern, *and* registered dietitian!

The Fine Print: The Application and Interview

If you are in a coordinated program in dietetics, then your didactic course work, degree, and internship experience are integrated. The student in a CPD does not apply for the dietetic internship because it's already a part of the program. However, if you are in a DPD, once you have spent time looking into potential programs and deciding what is right for you, it's time to put together your application. Prepare yourself. This is where the fun begins! The application process is partly fun, partly challenging, and partly anxiety-provoking.

Start early and give yourself enough time to complete your applications on time. Typically, applications are due in early February of the year you plan to intern. For example, if you're looking to begin a program in the fall, your application materials need to be finalized and shipped by February of that year.

You should start working on your application for internships at least six months before the computer match dates, which are in April and November. While some DIs participate in the November computer match, most participate in the April match. Setting aside enough time to complete the applications without any errors or typos is essential. When applying to multiple internships, it is helpful to develop a system for keeping the information from each school separate.

A new computerized application process, Dietetic Internship Centralized Application System (DICAS), was tested for the April 2010 computer match. Instead of applying to individual programs, prospective DI students completed one application, submitted one set of transcripts, and paid a fee electronically to cover the application cost for the DI program they hoped to attend. The computer match process remained the same. The computerized application was a success, and it will most likely replace the tedious assembly of application packets.

Your program director will have more information regarding the application and computer matching processes. You can also visit the Web site of a program you are considering, to see whether it uses DICAS and whether there are additional application requirements. As part of the application process, you will also need to mail a copy of your official transcript from each college and university you have attended.

Some students apply to only one DI, while others apply to ten. Both approaches are extreme. Shooting for only one program reduces your chances of getting an appointment, and going for ten is very expensive. Instead, pick a happy medium. While one candidate may apply for four programs, another might apply for three. Just keep in mind that you will not get accepted to all four programs (or however many you apply to); see #7 in "An Applicant's Overview" (page 45).

You'll want to request transcripts early. The application itself has a place for grades, and you may discuss grades in your letter. However, the committee will require an official transcript. Most transcripts can be obtained from the university registrar's office for a nominal fee.

An Applicant's Overview

Here's a list of tips to help you stay on track as you make your way through the application process for a DI.

1. Check **application requirements** for each internship program. Determine whether the program uses the Dietetic Internship Centralized Application System (DICAS). Also check to see whether the program has additional requirements, such as an essay that you submit directly to the program.

2. Include **writing samples** requested by the program, which could be in the form of a letter of application, personal statement, or responses to specific questions about ethical dilemmas, clinical nutrition, food science, work-related scenarios, and so forth. These will be opportunities to show that you can communicate well and know your stuff.

3. Follow the instructions for the **declaration of intent to complete** or **verification statement**. (See box on page 44.)

4. Secure strong **letters of recommendation**. Consider your academic adviser, clinical nutrition professor, food management professor, DPD director, or employment or volunteer supervisor. Ask potential reference providers whether they are comfortable providing you with a great recommendation. That type of question doesn't put anyone on the spot and means you'll be more likely to get what you ask for—great references! It never hurts to approach the person a few months in advance. You want to avoid waiting a week before the applications are due. Professors, employers, volunteer supervisors, and others who could serve as a reference are

---

Verification Statements and Declarations of Intent to Complete

A *verification statement* form is signed by your program director only after you have successfully completed all DPD requirements and fulfilled your university or college requirements for graduation (that is, you've paid all tuition, fees, fines, and other bills and met all university/college educational requirements). If you are in your last semester of DPD course work when you apply to DIs, you will need to include a *declaration of intent to complete* form in your DI application, rather than a verification statement, and then follow up with a verification statement before starting the internship. Your program director is aware of these requirements and should work with you to provide the appropriate forms.

There are special requirements for students whose degree is from a college or university outside of the United States. Visit the Student Center of the ADA Web site (www.eatright.org /students) for more information.

quite busy. Give them plenty of time to craft a letter that will serve you well. It is wise to give them at least a month's notice; be prepared to provide details about yourself, such as a bio, resume, and suggested highlights.

5. Have **official sealed transcripts** from each school you attended sent to the DICAS address. This can often take a few weeks.

6. Take the **Graduate Record Examination** (GRE; www.ets.org/gre) if you're applying for graduate degree programs. If you're filling out a separate application to the graduate program, it may require you to submit your GRE results. Allow plenty of time to sit for the GRE and for your scores to be processed. You may also wish to allow enough time to sit for the exam more than once.

7. **Register for computer matching** on the American Dietetic Association (ADA) Dietetic Internship page of the D&D Digital Web site (https://www.dnddigital.com/ada/index.php). Currently, CADE works with D&D Digital to facilitate the matching process. The registration fee in 2011 was $50. Most programs use a computer matching

Hot Tip for DI Applicants

Apply to more than one program to increase your chances of getting appointed to an internship. Students who apply to only one program limit their opportunities. If there's truly only one program you can possibly attend, you should make an appointment with that program. Visit the director, tour the facility, and let the key players know who you are. This *may* boost your chances of getting in. Alternatively, you may discover the program isn't a good fit for you after your site visit. Some programs even have formal open house events or offer individual facility tours. But don't feel like you must visit every program, and note that a visit won't guarantee you admission.

system in which an applicant is matched to the highest-ranking program that offers an applicant a position. How are programs ranked? They're ranked by you, the applicant, based on your priorities. (If your employer is also your DI sponsor, you may not need to be matched by computer.) You only get matched with one program, which you then decide to accept or decline. Declining means you've thrown away your shot, at least this time around. It is extremely important that you only apply to those internships to which you are willing to accept an appointment.

8. **Prepare for your interview**, if applicable. Conference calls are usually used when travel is either impractical or too expensive.

Ranking Your DI Choices

Not sure how to rank the programs? It's best to put your number-one choice first. This choice should be a program you're 100 percent interested in attending and in a location you're willing to live. However, it may also be wise to consider the likelihood of being accepted to the program. Ranking is very important, and it is important to consider your qualifications and those of applicants accepted in previous years.

The Application

The application process will make more sense to you when you review an actual application. You can order the standardized application form from the Dietetic Educators of Practitioners dietetic practice group (www.depdpg.org). This application asks for several pages of information. It's almost like your life story condensed to include educational accomplishments, work and volunteer experiences, and honors. The first part is basic contact and education information. Then it moves on to names of your references, extracurricular activities, honors, grades, paid work experiences, volunteer activities, and course work. In addition, each application is usually accompanied by a cover letter.

The standardized application is accepted by many programs, although some schools may use their own applications. Do not let that confuse you. Applications will largely ask for similar information. Focus on reading the instructions for each school and then following them closely. Applicants should contact the DI programs to which they plan to apply for information on each individual program's application process.

A Word about Grades

Grades from college and graduate school are important. You can see from the application that program selection committees will want to evaluate your grades, and having good ones helps boost your chances of getting an appointment. However, your application will also be evaluated for extracurricular activities, letter of intent, and letters of recommendation.

Let's say you received two Cs during your first semester of college. Do not despair. Simply address the issue and explain how you corrected the problem; you can discuss the issue during your interview, if applicable, or in your personal statement. Maybe you hadn't developed your time-management skills, or living in the dormitory your first year was too distracting, but then you started keeping a personal organizer or you spent more time studying in the library. Use your subsequent grades to substantiate any claims you make. The point is to reassure committee members reviewing your application that you will excel in their demanding program. Illustrate that you are a performer and that your potential is great. They want to train someone who will succeed.

THE COVER LETTER

The cover letter is a key component of your application. This single tool shows selection committee members how you stack up as a communicator. We've seen a substantial number of letters over the years—some good, some less poignant. Brainstorm your ideas with a family member or friend. Push yourself to go for the uncommon, the extraordinary, something that will set you apart from the pack. The first paragraph should inspire the reader to continue reading to see how

---

Great Openings for a Letter

Here are two beginnings to application letters that illustrate what we mean by creating a letter that speaks for you.

Opening 1: "During your visit to the University of Hawaii last fall, I had the pleasure of hearing you address the issue of genetic engineering and the future of the human genome project."

This introduction shows you have proven your interest in the program director by attending her lecture at your school. Mentioning this in the letter helps build a connection.

Opening 2: "Each cigarette reduces life expectancy by seven minutes. But what about each added pound of body fat over ideal body weight?"

This opening could allow you to explain your interests in laboratory or clinical research. Perhaps you have plans to earn a doctoral degree in research and conduct research once you have your RD credential.

---

amazing you are. Do not waste your shot describing a medical problem, how you've wanted to be a health professional since childhood, or that you like to take care of people. Everyone says that! You aren't everyone. Use this opportunity to your advantage.

PROOFREADING

When you are finished with your application and your letter, triple check everything. Make sure there are no typos. Ask a friend to proof your application and letter for you. Pick the toughest critic you know and offer to pay a sum for every error she or he finds. This is your incentive to produce good copy and your friend's incentive to actually invest time proofing. We call this trick a win-win! Even though you have to shell out some cash for errors, it's best that your friend identify them before your applications go out.

Some folks accidentally send applications and/or letters to the wrong schools. For example, someone may apply to program A, program B, and program C. This student will go through and complete the application and the letter for program A, and while in a rush, print out two more copies and mail them out to programs B and C without changing the salutation or any other information specific to the different programs. As you can imagine, this does not leave a good impression!

A Closer Look

Internship Director's Corner

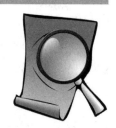

An Interview with Anne Brezina, MEd, RD,
the James A. Haley Veteran's Hospital Dietetic
Internship, Tampa, Florida

Kyle and From your perspective as an internship
Milton: director and practitioner of nutrition, describe the most important thing applicants need to know about dietetic internships.

Anne: I think that one of the most important things a prospective dietetic intern should know is whether the program they intend to apply for is a good match for them. A good example would be the applicant who already knows she wants a career in the area of pediatrics or community nutrition and working with women, children, and families. This person would not be a good fit for a Veterans Administration program, for example, where the population is largely males older than 50. However, for the applicant who wants a solid generalist experience, a VA program would be an excellent way to explore a sampling of core competencies and make a career choice after the internship.

K & M: Is there something that would help students while applying?

Anne: Avoid the stresses of waiting until the last minute to pull this complex application process together. Every program has specific requirements for the application, but most are going to entail getting official transcripts, letters of recommendation, and personal letters that ask for slightly different information. All of this will entail *time,* often utilizing the U.S. postal system, getting busy people to respond to your requests for letters of recommendation, and so on. It's predictable that everything won't fall according to your individual time frames when you are forced to work through university systems and relying on other people to come through for you. Start early!

K & M: Think of the top 10 applicants you ever admitted to your internship program. What stands out most about them?

Anne: We always look for the well-rounded candidate who has done an interesting sampling of everything. Although grade point average is important and is probably the single best indicator of accomplishment in a new graduate, it is not the only thing that matters. We look at paid as well as volunteer experience. Particularly, we are impressed with volunteer experience where the applicant has assumed a leadership role, not merely a name on a membership roster. We look for sincerity in the personal letter and actually deduct points from the candidate who is obviously inflating goals to impress the selection committee. Some of our most successful interns and former graduates have not been the ones with the highest grade point average, though.

K & M: Anything else you wish to add?

Anne: Unless they are a "perfect 10" who will successfully get into any program of choice, potential applicants should submit their applications to a realistic array of programs. I wouldn't recommend placing all their eggs in one basket and only applying to the one program where they absolutely would like to go. Pick one at the top of your list, one somewhere in the middle, and one "sure bet," if possible. This is practical insurance against heartbreak on notification day.

The Interview

Many dietetic internships require an interview. If the program requests an interview appointment, consider this a plus. The committee is interested in you as a candidate and wants to compare you further with other top candidates. Pick a date and time that suits your schedule and theirs. If you do not think clearly on Mondays or if you're brain is shot by the late afternoon, try to avoid these times. When asked about your availability, be specific and offer a few options, taking into consideration that you may need a day or two to prepare. Pull together work samples and your resume, and take time to practice your answers to potential questions.

The interview could go a number of different directions, but it is likely to begin with "So, tell us a little bit about you." This request is synonymous with the two-minute drill: you have two minutes or less to tell the interviewer your life story. Hit the high points: education, achievements, background, and where you're headed. Mentally picture your resume and use this image to feed your brain during the drill. Practice out loud with a friend—what you think takes two minutes may actually be five. Nailing this exercise will pave the way for a smooth interview. Another common line of questioning is about strengths and weaknesses. Be prepared. Turn weaknesses into something positive. Again, practice out loud, and polish your answers.

Interviewing is intense for both the candidates and the interviewers, so do not be surprised if interviews are shorter than you expect. Aim to control the factors you can—answer questions fully and confidently; be comfortable pausing for a few seconds after a tough question or asking to come back to it in a minute; and come in with your own questions, such as "What different patient populations would I have the opportunity to serve?"

Financial Aid Considerations

Being accepted into a dietetic internship program is an important accomplishment. You may receive notification of acceptance by letter, electronically, or even by phone. After some well-deserved celebration time, the next thing you'll want to consider is how to pay for the internship.

Unless you choose to enroll in the U.S. military dietetic internship programs, which offer excellent compensation and benefits, most internships involve tuition and fees. In addition, you may need to

Know Your Interviewers!

Alex Pryzytycki had a telephone interview with a program in Virginia. Before the interview, he rehearsed his two-minute drill, had an extra copy of his resume handy, and collected samples of some of his best work from school for easy reference. Despite all this and the interviewing preparation he did the days before, Alex still felt he didn't do that well in the interview. Why? He was on a conference call with five interviewers, and it was difficult to keep names straight. The whole process was intimidating. **The lesson:** Do not let the same thing happen to you. When you are asked for an interview—whether it's on the phone or in person—find out the number of participants and their names and titles in advance. You'll be better prepared the day of the interview.

cover housing, utilities, transportation, food, books and supplies, and entertainment. Most programs offer a list of required and recommended gear, including a computer, diet analysis software, textbooks, manuals (such as food-drug interaction and laboratory value guides), calculator, binders, and so forth. Our philosophy on this matter is simple: get the best your money can buy while sticking to your budget.

You may also need to purchase liability insurance. Some schools require interns to take out a policy. Ask your program director for recommended providers. Thankfully, this expense is relatively affordable and usually costs less than $50 for a year of coverage.

Sources of Financial Aid

Because it is very unlikely that you'll have the time to work during your internship (and working is strongly discouraged), you'll want to look into other ways of funding your unpaid time in the DI. Besides funding your own way, there are other options, including scholarships and loans. Speak with your college program adviser and director about some of these possibilities. The American Dietetic Association Foundation (ADAF), for example, raises millions of dollars to support dietetics education, including internships. Scholarships from the ADAF are awarded competitively, and the typical amount is $1,000. In 2009, 88 scholarships were awarded to DI applicants.

Financial assistance is essential for many students enrolled in dietetics education programs. If this is a concern, ask about financial aid at your preferred programs and consider this when ranking programs during the computer matching process.

Detailed information about federal grants and loans administered by the U.S. Department of Education is available online (http://StudentAid.ed.gov). Additional sources include state higher education agencies and civic, professional, and community organizations or foundations. The financial aid office or administrator at individual institutions can also provide information about their own scholarship programs and private loan options.

Applying for Financial Aid

Students are strongly encouraged to apply for financial aid electronically. The fastest and most accurate method is to complete the Free Application for Federal Student Aid (FAFSA). Your information is transmitted directly to the U.S. Department of Education and eliminates the additional processing time associated with a traditional paper FAFSA. This process is quicker and better for both you and your school, and most schools recommend this method. For more info, go to the FAFSA Web site (www.fafsa.ed.gov) and make sure to apply as soon as possible.

A Closer Look

Forming RDs: The Value of Dietetic Internships

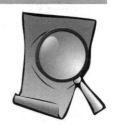

By Sari Budgazad

In light of contemporary nutrition issues such as weight-loss myths, lawsuits against fast-food chains, questionable herbal supplements, aphrodisiac foods, and revisions of the U.S. Department of Agriculture's Food Guide Pyramid, the need for RDs is apparent. In order to responsibly communicate messages of health and good nutrition to the community, nutrition students must obtain the RD credential by participating in dietetic internship programs. Currently, interns work in community, clinical, food service, and research settings in order to meet the criteria necessary to obtain the title of registered dietitian.

Internships approved by the Commission on Accreditation for Dietetics Education expose students to myriad experiences related to the dietetics profession. Brochures, Web sites, and promotional fairs help students find a dietetic internship that suits their professional interests. Once a student has applied, a computer-matching system determines where students will spend their next four to 24 months of training.

What is life like as a dietetic intern? Students enrolled in programs nationwide share personal accounts of their internship experiences thus far.

Many interns were lured into the field of dietetics upon realizing that they could make a career of the subjects to which they already paid a great deal of attention. "In college, I was mainly interested in science, but I have always loved food, exercise, and health," says Sarah Krimkowitz, an intern at Sodexo Healthcare Services, New York Metropolitan Dietetic Internship Program.

It was not until Krimkowitz enrolled in a dietetics program at the University of Delaware that she discovered nutrition is both a science and an independent profession. She admits, "It's a challenge because we work so hard to learn everything that there is to know about nutrition, yet the public believes what they want to."

When she becomes an RD, Krimkowitz intends to reinforce sound nutrition information. "In the broad scheme of things, I am interested in nutrition counseling and public policy making," she says. With six months of clinical experience under her belt, she appreciates the impact of nutritional care on various disease states.

Outside the clinical setting, Krimkowitz feels strongly about society's overindulgent eating habits. "Even a salad at a restaurant comes supersized and loaded with hidden fats," she comments. Krimkowitz continues on to her community rotation, committed to promoting the role of nutrition in preventive health. "Everything in moderation with regular exercise" is her message to the public.

In between classes, homework, and visiting patients, Krimkowitz makes time for healthy eating. After our phone interview, she politely excused herself to prepare a homemade pizza rather than calling for a lunch delivery.

Julie Oien, a dietetic intern from California State University, grew up participating in sports but also struggling with weight changes related to asthma. "Many experiences in my journey have prepared me for a career in dietetics," she says. Consequently, promoting body acceptance and encouraging healthy eating among children and teens have become her professional goals." An internship will make me more marketable as I enter a rewarding career in dietetics," she says.

The opportunity to work at a farmer's market and learn about nutrition outreach groups and resources represent only a few unique aspects of Oien's internship experience. "My interests have not changed during the course of a dietetic internship—only broadened my outlook," Oien says. She is an advocate for healthy eating, wellness, and disease prevention, reinforcing the fact that, "if you have just five minutes, you can eat healthy."

Karin Wirsig studied biology at Truman State University in Kirksville, Mo. "I was always interested in preventive medicine with a focus on wellness," she says. At the age of 19, Wirsig was diagnosed with type 1 diabetes. "I had already completed two years of premed requirements without fully understanding what it meant to be diabetic," she says. When Wirsig was referred to an outpatient community RD, she became motivated to take control of her health.

Through several counseling sessions, Wirsig learned to make nutrient-dense food choices and control portion sizes by keeping a food diary." Blood sugar control is like pushing on a gas pedal. Adjusting my insulin pump, counting carbohydrates, and incorporating daily physical activity is how I maintain a healthy balance without exceeding my limits," she says.

While pursuing an undergraduate degree, Wirsig was the cofounder of a diabetes support group. The group shared personal stories, discussed new research related to diabetes management, and participated in community events. During Diabetes Awareness Month, Wirsig helped a community service group initiate blood glucose testing for people interested in disease prevention. Coincidentally, Wirsig and her colleagues were served cookies, cakes, and soda as a reward for their efforts. "That was a good example of the difference between nutrition awareness and action," she comments. "Promoting good nutrition and healthy eating habits is easy. Sticking with it is the real challenge when living with diabetes."

Wirsig's personal experiences reflect her willingness to help others. "Doctors are the primary caregivers, but they often do not receive advanced nutrition education," she says. "This may influence the quality of nutrition care they provide."

As a dietetic intern, she devises and implements nutrition care plans for patients, whether it be calculating calories in tube-feeing formulas or conducting a Heartwise class to educate cardiac patients on healthy eating. Wirsig enjoys working in nutrition support, intensive care units, and pediatrics, which reflect the various clinical experiences offered through her internship at New York-Presbyterian Hospital (NYPH). Beyond providing direct patient care, Wirsig's true passion lies in research. "It is too personal for me to work with poorly controlled diabetics," she says. Wirsig would rather invest her time in finding a cure for diabetes. "More RDs are needed in nutrition research to shape Americans' eating habits," she says.

"I didn't know what a dietitian was until I was 19, during my sophomore year at the University of Florida," says Stacy Hammer, who recently graduated from Texas Woman's University Dietetic Internship. Hammer enrolled in college with the intention of becoming a pediatrician. "My classes always focused on treatment rather than prevention; therefore, I decided to look into a field that could prevent diseases such as cardiovascular disease and diabetes."

Hammer's professional goal is to equip people with diet and exercise knowledge needed to achieve healthy lifestyle management. "Prior to starting my internship, I had a good idea that I would not enjoy the hospital setting, and I was right," she says. "Establishing a relationship with the client was difficult to obtain in the hospital setting." Nonetheless, Hammer values her dietetic internship because it has enabled her to work at numerous sites in the community. "Being exposed to Dallas/Fort Worth Metroplex was a great experience for providing nutrition education due to its wide range of habitants. One week, I was working with families below the poverty line, and the next week, I was working with clients who owned private jets," she explains. Hammer also rotated at a food bank, where she distributed food, utensils, and educational materials within the community. She will be taking the RD exam this year and is pursuing a master's of science in exercise and sports nutrition.

Hammer feels that dietitians must expand the need for their services, despite limited funding for nutrition education programs. "Being an RD provides great job security because people have to eat," she comments. Hammer's nutrition message entails how to eat: "Life is about balance—it is not easy to achieve, but once achieved, being off balance is no longer an option," she says.

If life as a dietetic intern were a movie, Shannon Youngman would relate her experiences to the story of Erin Brockovich, the now-famous woman who uncovered the hidden truth behind a health scandal. According to Youngman, investigating dangerous weight-loss practices and bringing bad nutrition to justice is an essential part of a dietitian's career. "When I become an RD, it will show the public that I have completed a state requirement, and I will become a better resource," she notes.

Youngman is pursuing a dietetic internship at Oakwood College in Huntsville, Ala. Her professional goals involve earning the credential as an RD, certified diabetes educator, and achieving a degree in culinary arts. "I am interested in cooking because our culture has gone from home-cooked meals to meals on-the-go. I would like to provide a service that delivers healthy cooking to the on-the-go-family," she explains.

"I have always enjoyed working with children," Youngman says. The internship has provided her with novel experiences, such as working with children and families with disabilities. In addition to the Children's Rehabilitation Service of Alabama, she rotates at the Parkview Diabetes Center in Colorado, the Bessemar Dialysis Center in Alabama, Birmingham City Schools, and many other nutrition-related sites.

During the next few months, Youngman will continue to deliver quality nutritional care to diverse populations—largely Hispanic, Native American, and African American patients suffering from chronic diseases. "Credentials aren't just handed out; you actually have to work to earn them," she says.

Given society's surge of fad diets and nutrition quackery, dietitians are forced into an uphill battle to provide accurate information to the public. "However, with certification, nonlicensed nutritionists are held accountable for poor practices," Youngman says. Her nutrition message is: "Invest in your health—the future of good nutrition is a long-term investment."

Dietetic interns constitute a group traveling along a similar path, yet the road forks in many directions when they are asked about individual career goals. "My ultimate career goal is to become a certified diabetes educator, guide diabetic patients, and provide insulin pump therapy," says Amanda Murray, a dietetic intern, also at Oakwood College. While Wirsig may become a leader in nutritional research related to diabetes, Murray intends to build a career around diabetic counseling. Her professional goals stem from her personal experiences with diabetes management for 11 years. Numerous accounts with dietitians have been beneficial in helping her realize the importance of good nutrition for maintaining a healthy life. "Throughout my internship, I have been lucky that my preceptors have had enough confidence in me to help me plunge forward and counsel patients on their diets," Murray says.

Christy Youens, a dietetic intern at Texas Woman's University, realized the essential role diet plays in the pathophysiology of disease following her father's heart attack. Through her internship, Youen hopes to gain clinical experience and also work in a community nutrition education outreach program. "As clients encounter daily nutrition information, it is my job to decipher the truth of it all," she says. "Eat well, live well" is Youen's nutrition message to the public.

The RD exam may eventually blow over, but memories of the dietetic internship linger. Alan Lee, RD, CDN, CFT, still values his dietetic internship. "Being able to interact with an interdisciplinary health care team is helpful. The internship trained me to encounter professionals on a real level," Lee says. In addition to maintaining a private practice and expanding his role as a clinical research coordinator, Lee serves as the current president of the Greater New York Dietetic Association. "Registered dietitians are the nutrition experts. Make sure you have at least one yearly checkup with one" is Lee's nutrition message.

"I began the internship naive and extremely open-minded," says Meredith Liss, BS, MA, RD, CDN. "My interests were constantly changing. For example, after the endocrine rotation, I wanted to specialize in diabetes; after the renal rotation, I wanted to specialize in renal." Liss pursued a 50-week internship at NYPH and became exposed to all areas of dietetics. "I was fortunate to work with a variety of preceptors and dietetic professionals who all influenced me in different ways," she says. In fact, Liss currently works as a preceptor and outpatient HIV dietitian at NYPH. "Plan ahead. Don't be victimized. Empower yourself to make healthy food choices in all situations" is Liss's message to the public.

Dietetic interns receive a working education. With one foot in a classroom and one foot in a patient's room, they learn to apply textbook knowledge to real nutrition practice. The ingredients to a successful career in dietetics comes from blended experiences. Students are encouraged to interact with diverse populations. Advanced surgery, burn, cardiology, diabetes, enteral nutrition support, food service, and geriatrics represent a few areas along the alphabet of clinical disciplines.

Beyond the clinical environment, interns are exposed to a population whose lifelong food choices may be more sugar-coated than wholesome. "High-fat, high-cholesterol, and high-sodium foods are inexpensive and readily available to the public, contributing to obesity and other chronic diseases," says Jen Nelson, a cardiac RD at NYPH. As a preceptor, Nelson communicates to her interns that dietitians are continuously challenged to combat bogus nutrition advice. Nelson recalls the days when her grandmother kept countless jars of vitamins. "At the slightest hint of a sneeze, she would be at the ready with vitamin C—'have a chewie,' she would say." In response to the quick-fix mentality of popping dietary supplements, Nelson's nutrition message is "No magic pill will prevent or undo damage; being healthy is an everyday thing."

As dietitians-to-be, it is the interns' responsibility to not merely take note of but to actively get involved in nutrition issues encountered at the local, state, and national level. "If people learn to take everything they hear as a half truth," says Patty DeBari, RD, "then there is room for the dietitian to effectively correct nutrition fallacies and communicate sound information to the public."

"With the RD, you are viewed as more credible by clients and allied health care professionals. Without the credential, you are not held up to these standards and are likely to fall far behind," says Liss. The internship that leads to an RD credential is, in fact, essential to the growth of the dietetics field.

Reprinted from Today's Dietitian, *April 2003, pp. 31–32, with permission of* Today's Dietitian ©, *Great Valley Publishing Co.*

4

The Registration Examination for Dietitians

The day will come when you're eligible to sit for the Registration Examination for Dietitians (also known as the RD exam). And when it does, you should be proud of everything you've already accomplished along the way, including years of course work and many hours of supervised practice (internship)—all within programs accredited by the Commission on Accreditation for Dietetics Education (CADE), of course. In a nutshell, this exam is a rite of passage, after successful completion of which you will be recognized as a registered dietitian (RD).

This chapter will continue to provide useful information, guidance, and tips for you as you progress ever closer to your goal of becoming an RD. We hope this chapter helps you feel confident about the process and that you leverage the resources to successfully prepare for and pass your exam!

RD Exam 101

The Commission on Dietetic Registration (CDR) is the credentialing agency for the American Dietetic Association. CDR awards and maintains your RD credential and it contracts with ACT, an examination testing vendor, to administer the registration exams.

The Registration Examination for Dietitians is designed to evaluate an RD's readiness to practice at the entry level. You'll be tested on dietetics concepts, principles, and procedures, and you'll need to be able to decipher graphs, tables, and formulas. Questions may ask you to solve problems or make decisions. Questions can come from any of the five content domains in the following list, and they don't necessarily show up in content order. (**Note:** the content outline printed here is from 2006 and was current at press time; however, a new outline will be activated on January 1, 2012. Contact CDR for updated information.)

- Domain I: Nutrition and Food Sciences (12 percent)
- Domain II: Nutrition Care Process and Model—Simple and Complex Conditions (40 percent)
- Domain III: Counseling, Communication, Education, and Research (10 percent)

Official Exam Resources

- CDR distributes the *Registration Examination for Dietitians Handbook for Candidates;* available online from the products, services, and resources section of CDR's Web site (www .cdrnet.org).
- Contact CDR staff for information about the exam by calling 312/899-5500 between 9:00 AM and 5:00 PM, Central Time, Monday through Friday.

- Domain IV: Foodservice Systems (17 percent)
- Domain V: Management (21 percent)

Once your application to become registration-eligible to take the examination has been approved (a three- to six-week process; see the section titled "The Application Process" later in this chapter for more details), ACT will send you an application form for the examination. After you have completed the form and returned it to ACT with the examination fee, you will be sent an "authorization to test" letter, along with information about how to schedule a testing appointment.

How It Works: Computer Classification Tests

The days of pencil-and-paper tests are no more. Gone are long waiting periods for your results, too. Now the exam takes place on a computer. If you've taken the GREs, you will be familiar with the testing environment and the multiple-choice question procedure. You also must know that there is no skipping of questions to ponder and return to later. You must answer each question as it comes to you, and the computer will then offer you the next question. Items, or questions, are administered according to test specifications, in random order.

ACT testing sites are located on or near universities and community computer centers. You have one year to take the exam once you have become authorized. The exam is a computer-based multiple-choice test that you can take Monday through Saturday. If you need to take the exam more than once, you must wait 45 days in between test days and you will need to submit another application, along with the $200 application fee, to ACT.

Anatomy of the Exam

You will be given a minimum of 125 and a maximum of 145 questions, which includes 100 to 120 scored questions and 25 pretest questions that will not be scored. The 25 pretest questions are being tested for future exams, but you won't know which questions they are, so it is best to concentrate on answering all the questions as best as you can.

To receive a score, whether it's a pass or a fail, you must answer 125 to 145 questions. If you don't answer the minimum of 125 questions (for whatever reason), you will not pass the exam. Refer to the CDR Web site for details about the topics on the exam.

Contacting CDR

Commission on Dietetic Registration

120 South Riverside Plaza, Suite 2000 Chicago, IL 60606-6995

Phone: 312/899-0040 Ext. 5500 or 800/877-1600 Ext. 5500

Fax: 312/899-4772

E-mail: cdr@eatright.org

The Application Process

The application process for the RD exam starts with your DI or coordinated program in dietetics (CPD) director filling out an online form to notify CDR that you're eligible to take the test. When CDR has processed the information and your eligibility has been established, it will contact both you, the applicant, and its testing agency—ACT, Inc., of Iowa City, Iowa. If it is the first time you are eligible to sit for the exam (this will probably be most of you reading this book), good news: ACT will automatically send you a one-page application form, the *Registration Examination for Dietitians Handbook for Candidates,* and instructions for completing the application and submitting the $200 application fee. After being notified by CDR, it usually takes ACT one to two days to send materials out. If it's not your first time taking the test, simply request an application from CDR by mail, phone, or fax.

As part of the application, you will:

- Sign the following agreement that upon passing the registration examination: "As a registered dietitian or dietetic technician, registered, I agree to abide by the Code of Ethics for the Profession of Dietetics, and to hold harmless the Commission on Dietetic Registration, other RDs and DTRs, or CDR employees for their activities in enforcing them."
- Complete the application for the exam either by paper or on the Web, and contact ACT with any questions. ACT mails each exam candidate a paper application along with a copy of *Registration Examination for Dietitians Handbook for Candidates.*
- Fill out your name, gender, and contact information, where appropriate. Also, include your CDR/ADA identification number. If your name changes during this process, notify CDR in writing and send along a copy of the marriage license, divorce decree, or court order, as appropriate.
- Check the box that describes the *one* pathway that best explains how you met the eligibility requirements to take the Registration Examination for Dietitians (for example, a CPD or DI).
- Include your program code number (these codes are available in the CDR handbook), followed by the name, city, and state of your program. If your program code is not the CDR handbook, leave the area for the code blank but still include the name, city, and state of your program.
- Mark "yes" or "no" that you are giving ACT permission to release your score, by name. Examination scores of all program applicants will be provided to the program director for program evaluation purposes, regardless.
- Include the fee for the RD exam, when submitting the application to ACT.

- Check that your application is complete.
- When online registration is complete, you will be given links to a downloadable authorization to test letter, which you can print, and a list of test centers. You must bring this letter with you to the exam.
- For questions about special accommodations due to a disability and/or required documentation, refer to the candidate handbook.

Tips and Resources for Exam Prep

Test anxiety is common. Most of us have it. Solid preparation leading up to test day helps relieve some of the drama, and getting a good night's sleep the night before also does wonders. After all of the class and practice hours you've completed, a month of review and exam preparation is usually sufficient. It's a good idea to make a plan, however, and stick to it. For example, you might study online and

---

Want to Practice for the Exam?

The ninth edition of the *Study Guide for the Registration Examination for Dietitians* (September 2011) features 100 practice questions and access to an online practice exam, the study outline, a list of references, examination tips, and rationales for 15 to 20 questions. To purchase a copy of the study guide, call the ADA member service center at 800/877-1600, ext. 5000, or go to ADA's online catalog (www.eatright.org/shop).

Many other test prep books and courses are also available. To find resources that fit your needs, look for advertisements in the *Journal of the American Dietetic Association*, or ask your advisers or mentors for recommendations.

assign certain dates to review that material. If you need a deadline to help get motivated, pick a test date and create your study plan backward from the test date.

During the period before your exam, you may consider a review course. It can take away some of the work involved in preparing for the RD exam because it offers structured lectures, study materials, sample questions, and plenty of practice. Review courses are usually designed to help you focus your attention.

What to Do the Night Before the Exam

Stop studying. By now you know all you'll need to know for the test.

Relax.

Read a good book.

Do not worry.

Enjoy a good and nutritious dinner.

Get plenty of sleep.

Plan a nutritious breakfast.

Do not worry.

Watch TV.

Rent a movie.

Exercise.

Take a hot bubble bath.

Go shopping.

Call your best friend for a long chat.

Do not worry!

Test Day

Be well rested, eat a well-balanced breakfast, and allow yourself plenty of time to travel to your testing center so that you are not rushed. Arriving a little early is a good idea. Your examination confirmation letter from ACT will provide detailed directions.

Before the day of the test, prepare everything you need with you on that day. It is imperative to remember to bring a printout of your authorization to test letter and a valid government-issued photo ID. Without the letter and ID, you will not be admitted to the exam. You won't need a calculator; in fact, you're not allowed to bring in your own. However, a simple calculator will be provided for you by the test center staff.

Once you're seated at your testing station, you'll be given some time to get familiar with the computer process and review the instructions. If you need to leave the room in the middle of the exam, you

Situations That Cancel Your Right to Take the Exam

Once you've completed the exam, you're technically no longer eligible to take it again without reapplying. However, there are other, less ideal situations in which your eligibility can be revoked:

- It's been over a year since the date stamped on your authorization to test letter.
- You fail to cancel before the 2-business-day/48-hour deadline (cancel by calling the telephone number provided by ACT).
- On test day, you arrive late, don't present your authorization to test letter, or don't have a valid government-issued photo ID.
- You are caught cheating.
- You sit for the exam but then fail to complete it within 2½ hours.
- You abort the examination before it's completed.

If you need reauthorization, you'll have to get in touch with CDR to reapply, and you'll need to pay another application fee. If you need to do this, don't forget to include your name, reason for retesting, and your CDR/ADA identification number.

must have the proctor's permission, and you will not get that time back (you cannot pause or extend the testing time).

You have exactly 2½ hours for the actual exam, and the timer starts when you click on your first question. Remember: you cannot go back to review answers, change responses, or skip questions. It's a good idea to give each question adequate consideration before moving on. Also, recall that you must complete 125 to 145 questions for your exam to be scored.

You'll get your results following completion of the exam, and you can either leave happy or with a plan to take it again. A passing score is a score of 25 or higher (on a scale of 1 to 50).

A Note on Nutrition Careers That Do Not Require the RD Credential

The RD credential is widely recognized in the professional world, and if you plan to practice in a clinical setting such as a hospital or nursing home, you'll need to be an RD. The credential shows employers, health care professionals, clients, and patients that you've demonstrated competency in the field and that you meet certain requirements to practice.

On the other hand, a degree in dietetics without the RD credential may still offer viable career options. Some examples are work in food sales, public health nutrition, and foodservice management. Someone with a degree in dietetics, nutrition, or food could be a step ahead of someone who does not have this type of education.

5

Secrets to Success: An Orientation for the New RD

Congratulations and welcome to the world of being a registered dietitian (RD)! We know you have a passion for food and health, and that you've worked hard for the gold standard credential that assures the public of your expertise: the RD. In this chapter, we'll walk you through the one thing you must do to maintain your credential: continuing professional education (CPE). But we won't stop there.

We'll also show you ways to reach your full potential in dietetics by engaging with your professional organization and politics, as well as giving back to your community through volunteering and networking. Lastly, we'll take a look at what it takes to specialize, become a media expert, and publish articles in the media.

Maintaining Your Credential

Do you recall in Chapter 1, when we introduced you to the Commission on Dietetic Registration (CDR) as the credentialing agency for the ADA? Well, it's also responsible for maintaining your credential.

To maintain your credential as an RD, you must earn 75 hours of continuing professional education during each 5-year period.

Individuals who practice in the field of nutrition must prove they are competent to provide the services their jobs require. In addition to completing CPE credits, each RD must maintain a professional development portfolio (PDP) to demonstrate they are focused and capable of performing their duties. The PDP is an independent way to manage your CPE hours and is based on a learning plan that you design. Once you are a registered dietitian, CDR will send all the information you need to develop your own learning plan and manage your own portfolio. Such professional development is important because we know learning should never cease, especially in a field like ours where new research makes the headlines almost daily. Nutrition is a young science, and researchers are working constantly to add to the knowledge base. Sometimes, when new study results emerge with appropriate consensus, we change the way our profession does things. To know when to change practice, it's necessary to commit to lifelong learning and pursue continuing professional education. CPE and the portfolio help with the process.

> ### Financial Support for CPE
>
> The American Dietetic Association Foundation offers thousands of dollars to members to support education for students and professionals. The Karen Lechowich Continuing Education Award, for example, offers $1,000 to a new member of ADA (a member of less than five years) who wants to attend ADA's annual Food and Nutrition Conference and Exhibition (FNCE).

There are a number of ways to earn CPE hours. RDs may read CPE-approved articles or attend conferences, workshops, lectures, teleconferences, Webinars, and more. It's all spelled out in the CDR's *Professional Development Portfolio Guide*, which is available online from the CDR Web site (www.cdrnet.org).

Creating Your Portfolio

Developing the learning plan for your PDP takes five steps.

1. **Reflect.** Set aside some time—or several blocks of time spread over the course of days or even weeks—to reflect on yourself, your work, and your areas of strength and weakness, and then begin to establish goals for the short and long term.

2. **Assess.** Use the learning needs assessment worksheet that comes with the portfolio materials. The assessment walks you through the identification process to figure out which tools you will need to achieve the goals you set for yourself.

3. **Plan.** Next, once you have your goals in place and your learning needs assessment complete, create an actual plan. This plan will help steer you to specific activities (such as seminars, journal clubs, independent study, and graduate school) based on areas you identify, such as cancer, budgeting, human resource management, computer skills, writing and publishing, AIDS, and so forth.

4. **Implement**. As you attend professional activities and earn CPEs, document the CPEs in your activities log. This documentation will show you, your boss, the CDR, and state surveyors and regulators that you have been working toward building competence and increasing your knowledge base.

5. **Evaluate**. As you move through the process, the final step asks you to evaluate your learning plan. Take time to review

your accomplishments and see how you measured up based on the goals you set for yourself.

Then the whole process begins again. You'll know when it's time to create an updated portfolio because CDR will notify you based on your five-year reporting period. (Note that not everyone is on the same plan or cycle.)

You may feel a little overwhelmed by this process, especially if you're still a student or new graduate. That's perfectly normal. Our advice is to read the introductory materials CDR sends you that covers this topic and then call CDR staff directly with any questions, at 800/877-1600 extension 5500. If you'd like, you can get even more information from the CDR Web site (www.cdrnet.org).

Ways to Earn Continuing Professional Education Credits

One of the more popular ways of earning CPEs, according to our peers, is to attend conferences, workshops, seminars, and lectures. Topics are broad and include any number of areas, such as gastrointestinal health, money management, business plans, marketing, and thyroid disease. Whatever you're looking for, you can bet it's out there.

If conferences aren't your thing, don't worry. There are programs

Looking for CPE Events?

To find upcoming continuing professional education events you can attend, check out listings in the *Journal of the American Dietetic Association* and *Today's Dietitian*. Dietetic practice group newsletters also list events, as does ADA's Center for Professional Development (www .eatright.org/cpd). Another place that can keep you informed is the Professional and Career Resources section of the U.S. Food and Nutrition Information Center (http://fnic.nal.usda .gov).

Top Annual Conferences

ADA Food and Nutrition Conference and Exhibition
(www.eatright.org/fnce)

Clinical Nutrition Week (www.nutritioncare.org)

International Congress of Dietetics
(www.internationaldietetics.org/congress.aspx)

National Restaurant Association
(http://show.restaurant.org)

State Dietetic Association Meetings
(www.eatright.org/affiliates)

available on CDs and DVDs and via the Web. In addition, you can purchase audio of lectures or read books and self-study guides. Academic course work, case presentations, certificate programs, journal clubs, study groups, and professional leadership also provide CPEs. Just remember: the goal is a minimum of 75 CPEs per 5-year reporting period, although you may find it's pretty easy to earn many more than that. Check out listings for face-to-face and distance learning at the Center for Professional Development section of the ADA Web site (www.eatright.org/cpd).

Your Professional Organization: ADA 101

Many would argue that without a professional governing organization, a profession cannot exist. Your governing organization is the American Dietetic Association, which can provide intellectual

stimulation, motivation, and social activity for RDs while also pro-
tecting and promoting the profession. When asked to describe themselves, many high-profile and successful RDs mention they are members and leaders in ADA.

The American Dietetic Association is the national organization
representing over 70,000 food and nutrition professionals. We strongly believe in a unified voice for our profession, and we know the
best way to carry this voice is via membership in the American Dietetic Association. ADA, although large in numbers, is still composed
of individuals, and each one of us has a voice. We can each take part in
helping to shape what ADA is and what it will become. When something needs changing, one person can initiate change. When something needs sustaining, like the good work of ADA, many RDs can
maintain that work.

Did You Know Your ADA Membership Can Do That?

ADA offers members access to a valuable Knowledge Center.
Ever wish you had a research assistant to help dig up information on just about any topic connected to food, nutrition, and
health? Well, you do if you're a member of ADA. The Knowledge Center is a resource library with over 3,000 books and 150
periodicals and a staff of a librarian and RDs who are ready to
help busy students and professionals. Whenever you are pressed
for time or unable to find all the information you require, do
what we do—fire off an e-mail to knowledge@eatright.org with
your question. Most times, the Knowledge Center staff will respond within 24 hours or less, and they share a ton of citations,
Web links, and facts to answer your questions.

ADA includes groups by state or district affiliate, dietetics practice area, or special interest. Information about all these groups is also available online in the ADA Member Center (www.eatright.org /Members).

State Affiliates and District Affiliates

All 50 states, plus Puerto Rico, the District of Columbia, and the American Overseas Dietetic Association, have representation in ADA. The state or district level is synonymous with the affiliate level, so keep that in mind if you hear either term used.

When you become an ADA member, you are automatically part of your own state's affiliate group; however, if you prefer to be a member of another state association, you can. Let's say you are originally from Arkansas and you worked there for 10 years, then you moved to Washington, DC. You have the option of joining your new affiliate (DC) or remaining part of your former affiliate (Arkansas).

For more information on ADA's 53 affiliate (state and district) associations, annual meeting dates, district dietetic associations, and job lines, contact the respective affiliate offices or visit their Web sites. Contact information for all affiliates is available in the ADA Member Center (www.eatright.org/affiliates).

Dietetic Practice Groups (DPGs)

ADA brings together individuals who are food and nutrition professionals: DTRs, foodservice administrators, chefs, clinical dietitians, community nutrition professionals, students, clinical researchers, educators, consultants, entrepreneurs, and beyond. As you can see, this short list is quite diverse. Once in ADA, members may find it more beneficial to network with others who have similar career interests and skills. To locate people who work in weight management, for example, you can become a member of ADA's Weight Management dietetic practice group. Of course, that's only one of a possible 28 groups you could join! There's no limit, and many practitioners belong to two or more DPGs.

Besides networking opportunities, DPGs host educational conferences and publish newsletters to keep members informed of developments in the field that could alter practice and improve delivery of services to clients. DPGs also give members an opportunity to get involved on a national and local level by running for elected office or serving on committees. Furthermore, DPG members contribute to ADA projects and legislative initiatives, author books, and create educational videos, and they work on position papers.

Whenever you pay your ADA membership dues, you can also join DPGs. The membership term is the same for ADA and DPGs. DPG membership expenses may be considered business related. Check with a tax professional to determine what can be used for a tax deduction.

Member Interest Groups

ADA currently has seven member interest groups designed to promote diversity and networking within the profession. These are:

- Chinese Americans in Dietetics and Nutrition
- Fifty Plus in Nutrition and Dietetics
- Filipino Americans in Dietetics and Nutrition
- Latinos and Hispanics in Dietetics and Nutrition
- Muslims in Dietetics and Nutrition
- National Organization of Blacks in Dietetics and Nutrition
- National Organization of Men in Nutrition

Learn more about any of these special interest groups at the ADA Member Center (www.eatright.org/migs).

Which DPGs Are Right for You?

Information about ADA's 28 dietetic practice groups can be found in the Member Center section of ADA's Web site (www.eatright.org/dpgs).

- Behavioral Health Nutrition
- Clinical Nutrition Management
- Diabetes Care and Education
- Dietetic Educators of Practitioners
- Dietetic Technicians in Practice
- Dietetics in Health Care Communities
- Dietitians in Business and Communications
- Dietitians in Integrative and Functional Medicine
- Dietitians in Nutrition Support
- Food and Culinary Professionals
- Healthy Aging
- Hunger and Environmental Nutrition
- Infectious Diseases Nutrition
- Management in Food and Nutrition Systems
- Medical Nutrition Practice Group
- Nutrition Education for the Public
- Nutrition Educators of Health Professionals
- Nutrition Entrepreneurs
- Oncology Nutrition
- Pediatric Nutrition
- Public Health/ Community Nutrition
- Renal Dietitians
- Research
- School Nutrition Services
- Sports, Cardiovascular, and Wellness Nutrition
- Vegetarian Nutrition
- Weight Management
- Women's Health

Did You Know Your ADA Membership Can Do That?

Your ADA membership offers you the opportunity to be listed in the National Nutrition Network/ADA Referral Service, which is helpful for those in the consulting business or private practice. Perhaps you want to promote your consulting business to canned good manufacturers, or you wish to mention your hospital's outpatient clinic as part of your community marketing plan. Members can sign up by calling 800/877-1600 extension 5000. Individual consumers and companies who need your services can search by specialty and state from the ADA Web site (www.eatright.org).

Other Nutrition Organizations

Many RDs hold more than one professional association membership. ADA membership is popular for most in the field because it supports the primary functions of dietitians. As RDs begin to find their niche, they may find value in joining additional complementary organizations, such as the following:

- **American Association of Diabetes Educators** (www.aadenet.org)
- **American Society for Nutrition** (www.nutrition.org)
- **American Society for Parenteral and Enteral Nutrition** (www.nutritioncare.org)
- **American College of Nutrition** (www.americancollegeof nutrition.org)
- **Dietary Managers Association** (www.dmaonline.org)
- **School Nutrition Association** (www.schoolnutrition.org)
- **Society for Nutrition Education** (www.sne.org)

Your Voice in Public Policy

Your voice as an individual and as part of ADA can make a difference. For example, an individual ADA member called the office of New York Assembly member Daniel O'Donnell to discuss licensure of food and nutrition professionals. He spoke for 15 minutes with a staff member, who asked tons of questions about the issue. The next day, the ADA member received a call stating that Assemblyman O'Donnell planned to support licensure in New York. A few days later, the ADA member received a letter signed by Assemblyman O'Donnell with all the highlights of the phone conversation, and the letter reiterated that he would support licensure. That was one more lawmaker supporting our cause, and it only took a 15-minute phone call.

A Candid Guide to Volunteering and Networking

If you plan to enjoy your job, become successful, earn a respectable living, and connect with others, we strongly encourage you to get involved with volunteering and networking. You may have heard this already while in school or during your internship. We say "get involved" because we did, and we have enjoyed more opportunities because of it.

Volunteering

Getting involved means reaching out beyond your daily job requirements or schoolwork and participating and contributing to the food and nutrition community. You could become active at your district level (local association), affiliate (state association), or national association (ADA). You may even take part in the dietetics organization that's in your hometown or on your college campus. It does not matter which level you aim for, as long as you do something.

So what can you do to get involved? On the affiliate level, there may be opportunities to serve on committees, such as the public relations or newsletter committee. Some of your past professors may serve on the district association boards already, and you could ask them to help you get involved. E-mail the president or membership chair to find out if any committees are looking for additional members. We mention public relations and newsletter committees because both usually need assistance at varying commitment levels. If you can only spare two hours each week, there will probably be something that takes two hours to do; if you've got ten hours, there will be a ten-hour job. Count on it. Or perhaps you have a special talent for fundraising. Dietetic associations are looking for people to help raise funds for scholarships, political action committees, and conference expenses, among other things. If you enjoy your work on any given committee, consider looking ahead to a position as a committee leader.

These are only a few possibilities. Throw your hat in the ring with an e-mail. You never know how many doors will open down the road because of it, not to mention what you will learn.

Networking

As we have used one or two clichés in this text already, it won't hurt to use another. These days, and in this profession, it's all about who you know. Staying connected to others will keep you informed. You connect with others by volunteering for projects and dietetics-related events. Then when you meet people at one of these events or while working on the project, introduce yourself. It's easy, even if you are shy.

Balancing Work, Life, and Volunteering

Striking a healthy balance in your professional and personal lives is all about planning. Get a calendar, schedule book, or personal digital assistant and map out your days and weeks. Set aside time for just about everything. While it sounds a bit controlling, we assure you this sort of plan is the path to organizing your life and achieving success. Furthermore, once everything is laid out before your eyes, you can see where there's an extra 30 minutes or 2 hours to volunteer. You can also see when it's necessary to say no because there isn't a moment remaining.

Knowing when to say "no" is as important as knowing when to say "yes." No one knows your calendar and abilities like you do. It's fine to push yourself and be ambitious, but take care not to overdo it. Spreading yourself too thin, making too many commitments, or failing to complete tasks as best you can will make you look bad. When others are counting on you to perform, you should accept responsibility only if you know it's possible. Otherwise, pass on the opportunity, recommend names of a couple of other people who may be a good fit, and wait for the next time you can help. There will always be a next time.

Extend your hand and say, "I'm Olivia, and I'm a new RD." Then the people you are meeting will introduce themselves. After that, you should use about 10 to 30 seconds of information you have already prepared. It's not a monologue, and it's not an invitation to monopolize the conversation. Instead, it should be a moment where you can share some additional information about yourself, such as what you're working on or what you're interested in learning more about. Brevity is the order of the day, at first.

Your aim should be to learn something about the people you're meeting. Show genuine interest and try to make a connection, and look for ways you might be able to help your new acquaintances. Perhaps you'll meet a public relations chair who needs another volunteer. There you go! You just extended your professional network.

Networking is not about climbing some invisible ladder just to meet people and gain favors. Meeting people and doing favors for them is more like it. That way, when you need something, folks in your network are more apt to help because you have already confirmed you aren't just a climber but rather an important member of the professional community.

Looking Ahead: Specializing

After completing a dietetic internship and taking your RD examination, you are qualified to work as an entry-level practitioner. Once you get a few years of experience behind you—or if you already have an extensive history of advanced study—you may wish to pursue specialized practice areas. Most often, positions in specialized areas prefer or require board certification, such as the certified diabetes educator (CDE) credential or the certified specialist in pediatric nutrition (CSP). Once you meet all the requirements for application to a particular certification, you will take an examination. Not all certification programs require years of experience, so check with the board certifying agency. In addition, you may wish to pursue certification in exercise and training, health care quality assurance, or counseling. These activities can count toward your required 75 CPE hours.

Additional Certification Programs of Interest to RDs

The following programs are approved nutrition-related certification programs that can qualify toward your CPE requirements:

- **Board Certified—Advanced Diabetes Management**. American Association of Diabetes Educators and American Nurses Credentialing Center Commission on Certification, 8515 Georgia Ave., Suite 400, Silver Spring, MD 20910-3492. Phone: 800/284-2378; Web site: www.nursingworld.org/ANCC.
- **Certified Diabetes Educator.** National Certification Board for Diabetes Educators, 330 East Algonquin Road, Suite 4, Arlington Heights, IL 60005. Phone: 847/228-9795; fax: 847/228-8469; Web site: www.ncbde.org.
- **Certified Nutrition Support Clinician.** National Board of Nutrition Support Certification, Inc., 8630 Fenton St., Suite 412, Silver Spring, MD 20910. Phone: 800/727-4567, 301/587-6315; fax: 301/587-2365; e-mail: aspen@nutr.org; Web site: www.nutritioncare.org.
- **Certified Personal Trainer.** National Council on Strength and Fitness, 1320 S. Dixie Hwy, Suite 910, Coral Gables, FL 33146. Phone: 800/772-6273; fax: 305/666-4622; e-mail: info@ncsf.org; Web site: www.ncsf.org.
- **International Board Certified Lactation Consultant.** International Board of Lactation Consultant Examiners, 6402 Arlington Blvd., Suite 350, Falls Church, VA 22042. Phone: 703-560/7330; fax: 703/560-7332; e-mail: iblce@iblce.org; Web site: www.iblce.org.

(continued)

Additional Certification Programs of Interest to RDs
(*continued*)

- **ACE-Certified Clinical Exercise Specialist, ACE-Certified Group Fitness Instructor, Lifestyle & Weight Management Coach Consultant, ACE-Certified Personal Trainer.** American Council on Exercise, 4851 Paramount Drive, San Diego, CA 92123. Phone: 888/825-3636; Web site: www.acefitness.org.
- **ACSM Certified Personal Trainer, ACSM Health/Fitness Instructor, ACSM Health/Fitness Director, ACSM Exercise Specialist, or ACSM Program Director.** American College of Sports Medicine, P.O. Box 1440, Indianapolis, IN 46206-1440. Phone: 317/637-9200; fax: 317/634-7817; e-mail: crtacsm@acsm.org; Web site: www.acsm.org.
- **Certified in Family and Consumer Sciences.** American Association of Family and Consumer Sciences, 400 N. Columbus St., Suite 202, Alexandria, VA 22314. Phone: 703/706-4600, 800/424-8080; fax: 703/706-4663; e-mail: info@aafcs.org; Web site: www.aafcs.org.
- **Certified Health Education Specialist.** National Commission for Health Education Credentialing Inc., 1541 Alta Drive, Suite 303, Whitehall, PA 18052-5642. Phone: 888/624-3248; fax: 800/813-0727; e-mail: nchec@nchec.org; Web site: www.nchec.org.
- **Certified Professional in Healthcare Quality.** Healthcare Quality Certification Commission, National Association for Healthcare Quality, 470 W. Lake Avenue, Glenview, IL 60025. Phone: 800/966-9392; Web site: www.nahq.org.

(*continued*)

(continued)

- **Certified Strength and Conditioning Specialist or NSCA-Certified Personal Trainer.** National Strength and Conditioning Association Certification Commission, 1885 Bob Johnson Drive, Colorado Springs, CO 80906. Phone: 800/815-6826; Web site: www.nsca-cc.org.
- **Certified Personal Trainer.** National Academy of Sports Medicine. Phone: 800/460-6276; Web site: www.nasm.org.
- **National Certified Counselor.** National Board for Certified Counselors, 3 Terrace Way, Suite D, Greensboro, NC 27403. Phone: 336/547-0607; fax: 336/547-0017; e-mail: nbcc @nbcc.org; Web site: www.nbcc.org.

CDR offers the following specialist board certifications, which recognize that an individual has documented practice experience and passed an examination in a specialty area:

- Board Certified Specialist in Gerontological Nutrition (CSG)
- Board Certified Specialist in Sports Dietetics (CSSD)
- Board Certified Specialist in Pediatric Nutrition (CSP)
- Board Certified Specialist in Renal Nutrition (CSR)
- Board Certified Specialist in Oncology Nutrition (CSO)

More information about CDR certifications can be found on the CDR Web site (www.cdrnet.org/certifications).

CDR also offers certificate of training programs in adult weight management and childhood and adolescent weight management. Given that roughly two-thirds of Americans are either overweight or obese, taking part in specialized training may help in your practice, particularly if you work in clinical or community nutrition settings.

According to CDR, the training programs were developed by registered dietitians, physicians, and other experts, and include topics such as case management, nutrition assessment, environmental and genetic issues, prevention, physical activity, and behavioral management. Participants receive substantial CPE credits toward their professional development. If you'd like to learn more about these timely programs, call CDR at 800/877-1600 extension 5500, or check out the CDR Web site (www.cdrnet.org).

Looking Ahead: Working With the Media

RDs have a lot to offer the media. You may see yourself as one day being an expert source for the media by providing quotes and interviews for magazines, newspapers, radio, and television. Or you may become a member of the media yourself by writing magazine articles, for example. Here's our candid look at working with or as a part of the media.

Imagine getting ready for work and the phone rings. It's a TV producer who needs you to come to the station in an hour for a live interview with the morning show host. This could be true for a spokesperson from the American Dietetic Association.

Journalists rely on the expertise of RDs all the time for interpretation of the latest research findings, tips on how to avoid weight gain after 40, and suggestions for lightening traditional desserts.

Next time you read *Shape, Fitness, Men's Health,* or *Prevention,* count the number of quotes you see from registered dietitians. If you live in a major metropolitan area, check out the nightly news health segments. Some are hosted by RDs, while others have RDs who appear as expert guests.

If you want to take part in the media, one of the best things you can do is to stay informed. Watch the local and national TV news, read newspapers and magazines, and surf the Internet frequently. Stay up on what's hot. This way you'll know what's on the radar of timely topics and what's important to different groups. You should also stay informed as a professional. Read peer-reviewed journals and subscribe to ADA e-mail updates, such as the *Daily News* or *EatRight Weekly*.

When the media ask to work with you, be sure you're ready for the job. Know your subject forward and backward, and stay focused on a few key messages you wish to convey. Tailor your message to fit the audience by making it relevant to them. It should be clear that you understand precisely what they need to know. Remember to give concise answers to the questions. Sometimes we know so much information we feel compelled to say everything we know, but that's not necessary. Journalists are looking for answers that are clear and to the point. Concentrate on "teaching points" rather than a lengthy discussion.

It's possible that an interviewer may stray from the subject at hand or ask additional, unexpected, and unrelated questions. Practice dealing with this and prepare a few statements that help get back on topic without seeming rude or harsh.

As you excel in your media work, you may find that you love it and decide to apply to become an official ADA spokesperson. Because the selection process is very rigorous and training is tough, you can rest assured that only the top candidates are selected to officially represent ADA members. If you are interested in this program, check out *Working with the Media: A Handbook for Members of the American Dietetic Association,* which is available online to ADA members in the Career Center section of the ADA Web site (http://www.eatright .org). Also, be sure to read about Cynthia Sass in Chapter 7.

Of course, you don't have to be an official ADA media spokesperson to get quoted. Go ahead and put yourself out there. Send your information to magazine and Web editors, and to TV and radio producers if you are skilled at doing live interviews. It may help to include a head shot (photo), resume, and biographical sketch illustrating your expertise and accomplishments in the field. If you're on good terms with a journalist, you may offer assistance by sending periodic e-mail notices of new research studies or reminders that you're available to help.

A Closer Look

Media Savvy Musts: Feel Confident at Your Next Media Interview

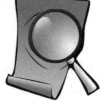

By Maye Musk, MS, RD

Believe me, there is nothing scary about a media interview. They just want your information. In all my years of being interviewed on radio and television, for newspapers and magazines, only once was a former friendly host hostile, catching me off guard. However, within ten minutes he was eating out of my hand. Keep to your facts, have a sense of humor, and you can handle any interview with ease.

The first time I was in the media was at two years old, when my adventurous parents moved from Canada to South Africa. I grew up with the media around our family as every year we went searching for the Lost City of the Kalahari in Namibia. My early experiences with the media were favorable; they were always nice and real people.

I started doing nutrition interviews as a student because my professor asked me to. She was nervous that she would be asked a question she couldn't answer. As a student, it didn't matter if I fluffed it. As it turned out, the questions were easy so I started off fearless.

This article isn't about marketing to the media but rather what to do if the media contacts you. The "musts" can be found in any media-training manual. These are the "musts" from experience.

Newspaper, Magazine, and Radio Interviews

- Return calls immediately. Deadlines for newspaper and radio interviews are very short, unlike magazine interviews, which have a longer timeline.
- If the media refers to an article or study, ask them to fax the article/study first and call them back when you have your facts in order.
- Prepare for the interview by asking a few questions: Is it live or taped? Who is the target audience?
- Research the subject, suggest questions, and add ADA info: to find a registered dietitian in your area, contact the American Dietetic Association at 800/877-1600 ext. 5000, or go to www.eatright.org.
- When answering questions, be honest—not perfect.
- Be prepared for disappointment. Interviews of four hours or counseling a magazine reader for three months can result in a one-sentence quote and not necessarily a good quote.

Television Interviews

When I gave "Media Savvy Musts," a talk for the Nutrition Entrepreneurs on this topic, I showed a tape of ten of my television interviews. I explained the advance preparation, why I chose to wear what I did, what was a surprise, and how good I felt afterward. Even though the edited tape contained the best parts of my interviews, the members liked to know I needed to prepare just like anyone else. These are my **Tips for Television Interviews**:

- If you knew all the questions beforehand and could edit the tape to your perfection, then your spontaneous interviews would improve. However, then they wouldn't be spontaneous, so do the best you can, and don't beat yourself up afterward.
- Although carefully worded and written facts sound better to your ear, spontaneity sounds better to the listeners.
- Check with the producer to ensure that your name and credentials are correct. Add MS and RD but not FADA, CDE, etc. MS, RD are confusing enough to the consumer.
- Use props. Don't be a talking head.

Spokesperson vs. Interview—Some Tips

- As a spokesperson, you will be media trained. This can be a harrowing experience, but it prepares you for the worst (which has never happened to me). It gets easier with practice.
- Food companies are not going to put words in your mouth you do not believe. They want the facts to be correct and for you to feel comfortable and confident with the message. Of course, if this is not the case, run.

- Unlike television interviews that are about your message, spokesperson work is about the company's key messages.
- Practice transitioning to your key messages when the host goes off the subject.
- Don't sound like you're advertising—your client doesn't want that either.
- "Desksides" means sitting at the desks of health editors and chatting about the product or program.

Appearance

- For phone interviews, pajamas are fine.
- For television: bold colors are suggested in every media-training manual. Patterns "dance" and distract. My "must" for women: wear a jacket. When they mike you, you don't need strangers wiring inside your dress/blouse.
- Look stylish. Enlist the help of someone whose style and taste you trust. I do.
- Avoid wearing large pieces of jewelry that will tap the mike or distract the audience.
- Make sure your hair is neatly arranged. You cannot believe how attractive, natural-looking wisps look messy on a closeup. For women, overdo your makeup; otherwise, you'll look washed out. The plus side is they're washing out your wrinkles as well. Men will need some powder; no shiny faces here. If there's a makeup artist, ask for a touch-up.
- Check under your shoes. Worn soles may show if you're perched on a chair.
- Look in the mirror just before you go on camera. A skewed tie or necklace is distracting to the audience.

The Interview

- Speak in short sentences (sound bites). (I still find that tough.) Answer the question directly then go into more detail.
- Look at the host, not at the camera, unless you are actually speaking to the camera.
- Show enthusiasm.
- Smile. Talk as if you are in your living room.
- Stay seated until they tell you to leave. You will notice when you watch television interviews that the host and guest continue talking while the music plays and titles scroll.

Afterwords . . . To Further Your Career

- Start a database of your television, radio, magazine, and newspaper contacts: name, company, address, telephone number, e-mail, what was said and done. You may need them at a later date.
- Send a thank you e-mail (unlike other contacts, mail is not popular at the news media anymore).
- Keep copies of all interviews and add to resume.
- Edit tapes.
- Laser copy articles and magazine covers. See how I've done it on www.mayemusk.com.
- Send me questions at nutrition@mayemusk.com.
- Enjoy, and keep our profession in show business.

Adapted with permission from Ventures *(Nutrition Entrepreneurs DPG newsletter). Vol. 18(2); Spring 2002: pp. 8–9.*

Looking Ahead:
Becoming a Published Author

Many major health and diet magazines and online publications have RDs on their editorial boards or have them contribute articles. This is a plus for our profession because it helps spread that word about our worth, and it's a plus for consumers because they get correct, scientifically sound information.

So how can you get involved? Study the publications you wish to write for. Examine their writing styles, the different departments, the types of feature articles they print, and review guidelines for writers. Most magazines and online publications provide tips and instructions to potential writers, and these are usually posted on their Web sites. Look for information on how editors like to be contacted (for example, e-mail versus surface mail) and how long you should expect to wait for a response after you contact them.

If you haven't published anything substantial up to this point, you may need to start small. Publishing in local newspapers or dietetics newsletters will get your name in print. Don't overlook local or regional magazines and Web sites, too. Most of these sources pay little or not at all, but what matters most is getting published samples of your writing (clips) to show future editors.

As you move up gathering more and more clips, query glossy magazines and major Web sites. Check the book called *Writer's Market* (Writer's Digest Books). It's published annually and gives information on editors and the magazines they work for. You can see how much they pay writers and what types of articles they are looking for.

Once you have identified a potential publisher for your writings and come up with an article idea, you're ready to make contact and find out whether the publication is interested. Editors are very busy. They receive hundreds of e-mails and letters weekly; sometimes more. Many of these communications are query letters, or pitch letters, presenting an idea for an article. This is how you should communicate, too.

Open your query letter or e-mail with an interesting fact or another attention-grabbing statement. This will make the reader continue with the rest of your message. Competition is tough and time is scarce. Editors can't possibly give the same amount of attention to every letter or e-mail they receive, so if yours is fascinating from the beginning you increase your odds of succeeding.

The next paragraph should explain precisely what you propose, such as a 500-word article on low-fat snack ideas for the magazine's how-to department. For this article you will rely on your own expertise as a food and nutrition professional, and you will interview a chef

Recommended Reading for Aspiring Writers

The business of writing takes a fair amount of study along with trial and error before becoming successful. There's also at least a hint of luck, if not more. Sometimes you may think there is no obvious method to the madness. This observation may be true. Besides following the advice in this chapter, you can find useful information on getting published in Chapter 11 of *Making Nutrition Your Business: Private Practice and Beyond,* by Faye Berger Mitchell, RD, and Ann M. Silver, MS, RD (American Dietetic Association, 2010), as well as *The Complete Idiot's Guide to Publishing Magazine Articles,* by Sheree Bykofsky, Jennifer Bayse Sander, and Lynne Rominger (Alpha Books, 2000). Online, check out FreelanceWriting.com (www.freelancewriting.com) for articles, links to publishers' guidelines, freelance leads, and more. If writing becomes a focus of your career, you may find a membership in the American Medical Writers Association (www.amwa.org) worthwhile.

instructor from the Culinary Institute of America. Saying this demonstrates you've given appropriate thought to the article and you know how it will unfold.

Once you've told the editor your plans, describe yourself. Explain your credentials, your work experience, and your writing experience (if you have any at this point). Make yourself sound like a star—and do so confidently. Editors can't waste their time on people who don't know what they want and don't say what they can do.

Then close the letter or e-mail. Provide complete contact information in the closing. It's acceptable to say you will follow up in X amount of time if you don't hear from the editor first. Keep in mind it may take one month and up to several months. This information may be provided to you in the writer's guidelines.

Be sure to provide two or three recent clips. If you mail your query letter, also include a self-addressed stamped envelope (SASE) so the editor can easily reply.

A Closer Look

A Juggling Act:
Profile of Leslie Bonci

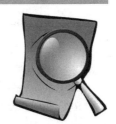

By Elise Chidley

A simple strategy for advancing your career and marketing your business involves becoming a nutrition messenger in many different venues. A dietitian in Pittsburgh, Pa., has done just that and has made quite a name for herself.

Leslie J. Bonci, MPH, RD, is director of the Sports Medicine Nutrition program at the University of Pittsburgh Medical Center Health System, where she lectures in the schools of dental medicine, nursing, and medicine. She's also nutritional consultant to recreational and professional athletes, including the Pittsburgh Steelers and the Pittsburgh Ballet Theatre. As if that were not enough, she's a regular speaker for corporate clients, a frequent guest on local and national television and radio programs, spokesperson for the American Dietetic Association (ADA), contributing writer to various magazines— and a marathon runner in her spare time.

Not surprisingly, Bonci's chief complaint is that there are not enough hours in the day. "There's so much I want to do that I'm getting to the point of thinking that I'm spread too thin," she says. "I'm not yet at the point of saying I have to let something go. Hopefully I'll be able to continue doing it all and doing it well."

Surprisingly, Bonci ended up in the field of nutrition by chance. As a high school student, she knew she wanted to pursue a career in the sciences but never thought of nutrition. Instead, she decided to study biopsychology. She found the subject interesting but was at a loss as to where it would take her career-wise. Once she had her BA, she decided to return to school and earn a master's degree in public health.

"While pursuing this degree, I took a course in maternal and child nutrition, and it was literally as if a light bulb went off in my head," she says. "I fell in love with the idea of nutrition and ended up doing my graduate work in nutrition epidemiology at the same time I was taking the undergraduate course I needed to sit for the registration exam [to become an RD]."

As Bonci comments, dietitians are all teachers, but, from the first, she has been involved in teaching large groups. Her first job as an outpatient nutritionist in Wheeling, W.Va., involved teaching classes for cardiac and rehabilitation patients. "I really loved the aspect of group participation," she says. After moving back to Pittsburgh, she jumped on an opening at the University of Pittsburgh Medical Center for an outpatient dietitian who would also have responsibilities teaching in the clinical dietetics and nutrition department; she has been teaching classes ever since.

She finds that teaching within the dental, medical, and nursing schools has its own challenges and rewards. "I think [these non-nutrition students] are blown away by the complexities of the field," she says. "They're surprised to find that [changing a patient's eating habits] isn't as easy as just handing someone a piece of paper and saying, 'Do it.' They learn that there's really a lot that goes into encouraging people to make changes. There's also a lot for them to learn about the preventive aspects of nutrition. For the most part, they are learning the reactive aspect: what to do after somebody has a problem. They've been extremely receptive to [the courses I teach]. They're realizing the lack of [nutritional] training in their own profession and they need to know this because their patients are asking about it."

Bonci developed her specialty in sports medicine in part because of her early participation in the University of Pittsburgh's wellness program, which is open to all students, faculty, and staff. "I would give lectures, and, as a result, a lot of athletes from the various programs would come and ask if I'd be willing to answer their questions. I started working with the Pitt athletic department and have been working with them on a regular basis for years."

It was through her work with the University of Pittsburgh athletes that Bonci was asked to be nutrition consultant for the Steelers. "One of the Pitt athletic trainers was a former student of the trainer for the Steelers." Bonci explains. The Steelers' trainer asked Bonci's colleague to recommend a nutrition consultant, and Bonci soon found herself working with one of the players. "The player was able to achieve some significant changes in terms of weight that impacted his performance." Bonci says. "Then I got a call from the president of the Steelers, saying, 'You're hired.' It's really wonderful to be able to do this."

Bonci began working with the Pittsburgh Ballet Theatre through her work with the children in the Ballet Theatre School, some of whom were suffering from eating disorders. "I thought it would be appropriate to come and address each and every class at the school, and a few of the dancers in the company were outside and just started peeking in and listening," she says. "Later I got a call from the director of the company asking me to please come and work with the dancers."

The challenges Bonci addresses among the football players are different from those that face the dancers. While the dancers are all anxious to keep their weight down, many of the football players are primarily concerned with bulking. "The underlying thread that ties all of these athletes together is the frequency with which they're eating, when food tends to be concentrated, and how that affects their performances," she explains. "Whether somebody is in the weight room, out there doing sprints on the field, or in the ballet studio for hours on end, they need to be as energized at the end of the day as they are at the beginning. So I look at food from the performance perspective and fine-tune [diet] to the individual body type."

With the football players, Bonci deals with issues like compulsive overeating, the need to gain weight, and unhealthy eating patterns such as only eating once a day. With the dancers, she runs into classic eating disorders as well as dehydration and a tendency to overdose on caffeine.

"Eating disorders are much more prevalent than they should be and are a major concern across the United States," says Bonci. "All the ballet companies are trying to address the problem. In and of itself, [an eating disorder] can be tremendously damaging for the dancer and may have orthopedic consequences, such as stress fractures, that can cause career-ending injuries. We're trying to prevent that as much as possible, but it isn't enough just to present the grim facts; you have to offer alternatives. Realistically, dancers are not going to sit down to a three-course meal, but they do need to know that there are many foods they can eat. Next week, I'm going to talk about particular foods that I think all dancers should have in their cupboards to keep them nutritionally in balance, healthy, and energized."

Long before her high-profile work with the Steelers and the Pittsburgh Ballet Theatre, Bonci was becoming known as a media dietitian. When she first started working as an outpatient dietitian at the University of Pittsburgh Medical Center, she was quick to respond to solicitations from the media. "There would be calls to the news bureau all the time from the local news station wanting someone to do nutrition stories," she says. "Obviously, no one was interested in doing it, or they were too scared, or whatever. I always enjoyed doing those types of things; so I started to do that very regularly. Then, when the opportunity arose to apply for the spokesperson position with the ADA, I jumped on it because I thought it would be really nice to represent the American Dietetic Association nationally." As a result of her enthusiasm for this type of work, Bonci has appeared on the "Today Show" several times for the Eat Smart segment.

Bonci says that while her media work has all been done on a voluntary basis without financial reward, she has gained much from it in terms of experience and self-confidence. The media training she received has helped her in her own practice and in the lecture room. "I can't put a price on it because of the benefit it has provided back to me," she comments.

In addition to writing for various magazines, including *Pennsylvania Health and Fitness*, Bonci has also contributed chapters to various textbooks, including two chapters in *Sports Nutrition: A Guide for the Professional Working with Active People*, edited by C. Rosenbloom and published by the ADA in 2000. She is currently working on a book to be titled Your Gut Reaction: A Guide to Intestinal Wellbeing [published by Wiley in 2003 as *ADA Guide to Better Digestion*]. Her interest in gastrointestinal health is long-standing and began when she was approached by the Intestinal Disease Foundation to put together an educational seminar for dietitians. She intends her book to be a practical and user-friendly guide for the consumer on everything from irritable bowel syndrome to Crohn's disease. She also has plans to write a general guide on sports nutrition for athletes.

Bonci advises young nutrition professionals to maintain a sense of humor in whatever they do. "It's very important not to take yourself too seriously," she says. "Humor really wins people over and helps them to learn well." She also advises her students to try to learn something new every day. "It doesn't matter how insignificant it may be," she adds. "Everything you do in your career will teach you something. You always need to figure out what you can learn in a positive way from your particular positions and apply it."

Reprinted from Today's Dietitian, *March 2001, pp. 24–25, with the permission of* Today's Dietitian ©, *Great Valley Publishing Co.*

6

Scoring Your First Gig and Beyond

Good news! Your hunt for the right dietetic internship (DI) has prepared you with skills that will transfer into the job hunt. You know how to research DIs (now, you'll be researching jobs). You also know how to ask for strong recommendations, prepare for an interview, and put together a winning application (now, you'll be polishing your resume, cover letters, and marketing materials). It may be a good idea to seek general guidance from your academic career center or a book dedicated to the topic. This chapter will assume you are already pursuing that general information and will instead mostly focus on information specific to the job hunt within the dietetics field.

After the sampling of practice areas you've had through your DI experience, you may still have broad interests in the field of dietetics. It may be challenging to narrow down an area of practice to pursue for your first job as a registered dietitian (RD). While it may seem overwhelming, our best advice is to take a deep breath, consider your strongest interests, and start exploring with confidence.

Where RDs Work

As you may recall from Chapter 1, about half of practicing RDs work in clinical settings. In addition to clinical practice, RDs may work in sports nutrition, culinary consulting, publishing, work site wellness, the food industry, academia, and many other fields (see Chapter 1). With an aging population, the obesity epidemic, and high rates of chronic illnesses, there is a need for RDs in a variety of settings.

Networking, Again

As you begin to explore job opportunities, remember that a large part of finding a job is about the people you know. When you talk to a friend who knows someone at Company W who knows about an opening at Business L, you may have an early shot at applying for a job before it's announced on job banks. This advantage may help land you the job.

At this stage, your network may include professors and internship preceptors, and the contact people they provide. Talk to people who are doing the kinds of jobs you find interesting. Ask them about the career path that led them to where they are, what a day in the life is like for them, and what skills or personality traits make them good at their jobs. The following "Closer Look" by Maggie Moon highlights various career paths in nutrition, and includes insights from RDs who love what they do.

A Closer Look

Opportunity's Knocking— Your Best Career in Dietetics Awaits

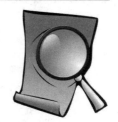

By Maggie Moon, MS, RD

Whether you're new to the field or firmly planted in your practice, you may wonder what else is out there—it's OK to be curious! Take our quiz, see how you rate, and get inspired by RDs who have found their ideal jobs.

Are you job curious? If you're like most RDs, there are about as many areas of nutrition that spark your interest as there are new products that hit grocery store shelves each year. According to the Bureau of Labor Statistics, the average American will have about 11 jobs before they reach the age of 42. So if you haven't already had a handful of different jobs in nutrition, chances are they may be in your future.

The years of academic and practical training we all go through mean we have the expertise to make a variety of jobs in dietetics viable, though some may be a better fit for us than others. As nutrition professionals, we have a "nice problem": we work in a growth industry that offers diverse ways to work toward the same goal of helping people eat right.

Whether you're fresh out of your dietetic internship, a few years into your first job, or a seasoned professional, you may be ready for something new—or perhaps just curious. Take the following completely unscientific ($P > 5$) quiz to determine what sort of career may suit you and read about how some of our colleagues are living their dreams.

Career Quiz

1. You're hosting a dinner party. You're most likely to:
   a. prepare longtime favorites you can trust will come out just the way you like them.
   b. strategically place finger foods and cocktails to get the conversation flowing.
   c. peruse the farmer's market the day of the event to grab what's fresh and let it inspire the spread.
   d. ask guests to bring their favorite foods, come up with a menu on the spot, and engage everyone in group meal prep.

2. It's a workday. You're most likely to start your day with:
   a. the breakfast you planned out the previous night.
   b. coffee or tea and a small bite.
   c. yoga or blogging.
   d. whatever you feel like.

3. When you started college, you:
   a. had your top three choices of dietetic internship programs scoped out.
   b. went to campus mixers to meet people who could help you and those you could help.
   c. joined a handful of clubs and had a crush on your smartest teaching assistant.
   d. founded a club and recruited members.

4. If you were a Microsoft Office program, you'd be:
   a. Excel.
   b. Outlook.
   c. Word.
   d. PowerPoint.

5. Your idea of a dream vacation is:
   a. a week in the Bahamas at an all-inclusive resort.
   b. joining an organized group trip biking across the Italian-French border.
   c. a "stay-cation" during which you finally cross off some local hot spots you've neglected to visit.
   d. finding a last-minute trip to Amsterdam and figuring out a place to stay once you've landed.

6. You have an important deadline coming up and you want to turn in your best work. Your first step is to:
   a. research what others have done in the past.
   b. gather the smartest people you know to brainstorm.
   c. start the process solo, culling down the list of great ideas you have at your fingertips.
   d. get started right away by yourself or with a team.

7. You see an abandoned mailman's bag full of mail on the sidewalk near your home. Your first thought is to:
   a. trust that the postman will return shortly and head home as planned.
   b. head home and call the post office and the police to alert them.
   c. scope out neighbors' mailboxes and knock on doors to determine where the mailman was last.
   d. look inside the bag for the mailman's identification information.

8. Your best feature is your:
   a. hair.
   b. smile.
   c. mind.
   d. hands.

9. If you were on a desert island and were allowed one magazine, it'd be:

   a. *Real Simple.*

   b. *The Economist.*

   c. *The New Yorker.*

   d. *Food & Wine.*

10. If you were a winter Olympics event, you'd be:

    a. cross-country skiing.

    b. speed skating.

    c. figure skating.

    d. snowboarding.

How You Score

For every "a" answer, give yourself 1 point. For every "b" answer, 2 points. For every "c" answer, 3 points. For every "d" answer, 4 points. Add up your points and match your total score to one of the four following categories.

10 to 14 points: You're a Steady Betty (or Bob)
Top five characteristics: responsible, organized, structured, perceptive, dependable.

In the workplace, you are perceptive and sensitive to how others are feeling and thrive on bringing structure and order to your world. Your great observational skills help you determine what people want or need. Your talent for organization helps you develop structured plans to help people reach their goals.

You may prefer stability over change and tend to be even-keeled. Being prepared and comfortable with your day-to-day tasks may contribute to your feeling of job satisfaction, and you may enjoy working in a setting that values your dependability and thoughtfulness.

If this sounds like you, you may be a great clinical dietitian, community nutritionist, or private in-person or telehealth counselor. It may be surprising to hear that the skills and temperament previously described may also come into play for a culinary RD working in an upscale Manhattan restaurant.

For Natalia Hancock, ACA, RD, culinary nutritionist for Rouge Tomate Restaurant in New York City, it's important to listen to customers and respond to their feedback, needs, and wants. And though she admits she is "always prepared for last-minute requests and meetings and it helps to be flexible," she still manages to take an impressively structured approach to her day.

Hancock shares what a day is like for her: She arrives at the Rouge Tomate office around 9:30 AM and checks e-mails, greets everyone in her office, and reviews the day's events with her interns. Then she heads downstairs to the kitchen and "pokes around to see what is going on in the kitchen with the chefs." Then she works at her desk either on material for articles, updating the nutritional charter, or analyzing a new dish from one of the chefs.

Her afternoon lunch is a working affair; she usually sits with a guest she has invited to introduce Rouge Tomate and its health philosophy. (She also trains the staff to discuss the restaurant's health philosophy with customers.) Over three courses, she jots down feedback for the chefs. After lunch, Hancock typically catches up with her inbox and e-mails the feedback from lunch to the chefs. Despite the natural ebb and flow of restaurant life—or perhaps because of it—she manages to create an organized framework for her day and loves what she does.

15 to 24 points: You're a Strategy Maven
Top five characteristics: strategic, future oriented, visionary, dislikes routine, has natural leadership abilities.

One of your professional strengths is that you can take in complex information and synthesize it to come up with theory-based yet practical and long-term solutions. In both your personal and professional realms, you enjoy being social, which makes you a natural networker and team leader. While you are part social butterfly/networker, you also need alone time to process information and develop those big-picture solutions. Your talent for thinking strategically applies to the work at hand and the arc of your career. You have no trouble seeing the possibilities down the road.

Your ideal work environment may be one that allows you freedom in your daily activities. You may make a great business owner, manager, supermarket RD, or consultant.

"Working in business and industry requires great communication skills and project management skills," says Annette Maggi, MS, RD, LD, FADA, senior director of nutrition at Nu-Val LLC in Braintree, Mass. She offers a few more tips for strategic, business-minded RDs: "You have to have fine-tuned experience in selling your concepts to business partners, be flexible, and be willing to play the politics game that exists in corporate America."

With a background in business consulting, Christen C. Cooper, MS, RD, who runs Cooper Nutrition Education & Communications in Pleasantville, N.Y., agrees that "knowledge of business and politics are huge boons to success in our profession, business in particular."

Cooper's must-have skills include the ability to read and write quickly and to analyze and prioritize tasks and information. She admits that she thinks she's a "right-brained person in a left-brain–dominated occupation." As an "out-of-the-box

thinker," she says, "this hasn't served me well in all environments. But as a consultant, it's a huge plus because nutrition
crosses over into so many fields that seeing the 'big picture'
in a creative way can differentiate you in the market."

25 to 34 points: You're a Jack (or Jill) of All Trades
Top five characteristics: project oriented, creative, broadly capable, excellent communication skills, independent.

Your professional golden ticket is that you are multifac-
eted, multitalented, and generally good at whatever interests
you. Your level of engagement in a project tends to be directly
linked to how much it captures your interest, which works out
well when you're very passionate about a project. (Read: Take
caution before accepting projects that may not keep your fire
burning.)

You also bring to the table a high degree of creativity, and
some may even describe you as an artist at heart. You're self-
reliant and independent, so although you enjoy working with
others, you may prefer to work alone. Your ideal work environment provides the personal freedom and space for your creativity and problem-solving skills to do their magic. Converse-
ly, you may dislike detail-oriented work or structured work
environments.

Your project-oriented, independent working style plus
your wide range of capabilities mean you have a lot of options. You may enjoy writing projects (e.g., articles, blogs,
books), developing recipes, or perhaps juggling 17 different
project-based consultancy gigs.

Every blog post is a new adventure for Jenna A. Bell, PhD,
RD, CSSD, blogger for Chicagonow.com/"Eat Right Around
Chicago." Armed with a laptop, a camera, and an empty
stomach, she explores how a dietitian with a great appetite
can eat well around the city. Bell shares that developing blog

posts requires creativity, humor, quick wit, and motivation. "I also have to be opinionated and find inspiration in a variety of nutrition topics to talk about," she says.

Cynthia Sass, MPH, MA, RD, CSSD, who is based in New York City, has no fewer than five major projects in her life at any given moment. She runs her own consulting company (Sass Consulting Services, Inc.), sees clients in a private practice, is a contributing editor and weight loss coach columnist for *Shape*, is a "food coach" to ABC News, and is a sports nutritionist for the Philadelphia Phillies and Tampa Bay Rays.

"I would say it's 50% nutrition related and 50% creativity, communication, and organization," says Sass. "In my experience, one of the most important skills in my day-to-day work is the ability to translate nutrition science into easy-to-understand, consumer-friendly terms."

"Whether it's with nurses or doctors, patients or family members, PR firms or journalists . . . if you can't communicate and connect, you can't do anything," says D. Milton Stokes, MPH, RD, CDN, owner of One Source Nutrition LLC, a nutrition counseling and consulting firm in Connecticut.

Stokes connects the dots. "No doctor will honor your TPN [total parenteral nutrition] recommendations if you can't communicate a rationale, and your boss won't give you a raise if you can't prove the justification," he says. Stokes also juggles being a media consultant, freelance writer (who recently came out with the *Flat Belly Diet! for Men*), and per diem clinical dietitian, all while working toward his doctoral degree in health communication.

"For my work, I must have solid skills in recipe development and analysis, writing, public speaking/media training, and a strong understanding about food," says Dana Angelo White, MS, RD, ATC, who runs Dana White Nutrition, Inc., in South Norwalk, Conn. She's also a sports nutrition consultant, certified athletic trainer, and culinary dietitian for the Food Network's "Healthy Eats" blog. She adds to her list of must-haves confidence, creativity, the ability to accept constructive criticism, and a sense of humor.

When asked about their "typical day," these Jacks and Jills responded (predictably) to the effect of "never heard of it." The type of work understandably varies day to day—from researching, writing, speaking, seeing clients, and developing or testing recipes to doing TV interviews.

35 to 40 points: "Action" Is Your Middle Name
Top five characteristics: entrepreneurial, self-motivated, hands-on, passionate, ambitious.

Your work is an extension of your values, and you wouldn't have it any other way despite the ups and downs. Your passion drives your professional choices, and you do what you love. Your ambition and charisma extend to your colleagues, and you enjoy mentoring others.

Because you're action oriented, you prefer practical tactics over theory. You're also highly creative, which makes you an asset when brainstorming. Not surprisingly, you learn best with hands-on training. Your best working environment gives you the freedom you need to do things your way.

For Ellie Krieger, MS, RD, *New York Times* best-selling author of *So Easy* and host of the Food Network's *Healthy Appetite*, being in the kitchen was always going to be a part of her career. She enjoyed exploring farmers' markets and being in the kitchen throughout college and loved exploring international cuisines, all from a personal interest that was eventually complemented with culinary school course work at the Culinary Institute of America in Hyde Park, N.Y.

"If you want to learn how to cook, get in the kitchen," she advises. "Formal culinary training is valuable, but even that means little if you're not getting regular hands-on practice in the kitchen."

Krieger also knew she wanted to reach people through the media, whether that meant writing, radio, or TV. She did the legwork and found her way into internships at CNN and a local CBS station. "Internships are critical," she says. She also interned with great mentors: Carolyn O'Neil, MS, RD, and Liz Weiss, MS, RD. "I said to myself, 'There's never going to be a *New York Times* wanted ad for the kind of work I really want,' so I made my own way into the industry."

Round Hole, Square Peg

Don't be discouraged if no single category describes you perfectly or if you find you are a composite of qualities described in more than one category. The consensus from colleagues in the field who love what they do seems to be that the ideal job is one in which your professional interests, preferred working environment, and skill sets all align. Notably, if it's just the latter that is lacking, there are options for getting up to speed through classes, internships, and work experience.

Get Inspired

Read on to gain inspiration from a selection of responses to the question, "Why do you do what you do?"

"I love taking my nutrition knowledge and breaking it down for real life. I find it exciting to bust myths, solve diet problems, and give advice that people can easily apply to their day-to-day life. I also love to eat, judge restaurants, and talk about them. I like any opportunity to express thoughts that make me laugh—I have a constant stream of jokes going through my head, and this provides me an outlet. Lastly, I have other jobs—and I do them from home—so this blogging gig gets me showered and out of the house to eat right around Chicago!" —*Jenna A. Bell, PhD, RD, CSSD, blogger for Chicagonow.com "Eat Right Around Chicago"*

"I don't think of what I do as a job. I really love this profession, and nearly everything I work on feels like a passion project!" —*Cynthia Sass, MPH, MA, RD, CSSD, owner of Sass Consulting Services, Inc., in New York City*

"I really love my job at Rouge Tomate. I get to use so many different skill sets and am so proud to be working with such talented and devoted individuals. I am able to promote the message of eating healthy from this position to people who really want to hear it. I am challenged every day. I am thrilled that nutrition and sustainability are part of such a chic and upscale restaurant. I feel good about collaborating with our chefs and creating healthy, well-balanced, nutrient-dense cuisine. It is a message that our country needs to hear." —*Natalia Hancock, ACA, RD, culinary nutritionist for Rouge To-mate Restaurant in New York City*

"Love it! The variety makes me crave more. Writing, teaching, advising undergraduates, working with patients— I get to do it all. If I am unhappy, I change my schedule or I create new projects. I do what I want to do. Having my RD opens many, many doors."—*D. Milton Stokes, MPH, RD, CDN, owner of One Source Nutrition LLC in Connecticut*

"I love my job because I work for myself. I set my own prices and I do my work my way. This autonomy doesn't appeal to everyone. But for entrepreneurs and those who just must 'do their own thing,' it's ideal. There are no guarantees

of money or success, but what you do you earn for yourself. You can feel especially good about your successes."
—*Christen C. Cooper, MS, RD, creator of Cooper Nutrition Education & Communications in Pleasantville, N.Y.*

"This is the job that is most aligned with my skills and talents. It's amazing to be a part of a start-up and have the opportunity to help shape our business and company."
—*Annette Maggi, MS, RD, LD, FADA, senior director of nutrition at NuVal LLC in Braintree, Mass.*

"Getting to speak to people who'd read my book and tried the recipes inspired me to get back into my test kitchen and start another book. I really feel like I know who I'm writing these books for." —*Ellie Krieger, MS, RD,* New York Times *best-selling author of* So Easy *and host of the Food Network's* Healthy Appetite

"I'm passionate about food and cuisine. I'm passionate about nutrition and health. I'm passionate about our environment and the climate. I firmly believe that if you have sincere passion for something, it will carry you farther than any other single trait. In fact, I truly don't consider all that I do to fit under the category 'job.' I'm on a career adventure. I love what I do for a living. It's a part of who I am . . . not just something I do for a certain number of hours." —*Jackie Newgent, RD, CDN, culinary nutritionist, chef instructor, spokesperson, and author based in New York City*

Reprinted from Today's Dietitian, *April 2010, p. 32, with the permission of* Today's Dietitian ©, *Great Valley Publishing Co.*

Where the Jobs Are

Part of the exploration phase is to get a good idea of the actual jobs that are out there. In addition to networking, browse job bank Web sites and the professional networking site LinkedIn (www.linkedin.com); and keep an eye out for Listserv job postings from your state affiliate, dietetic practice groups, or student groups. Web sites for local newspapers and Craigslist (www.craigslist.org) are also places to scope out potential jobs.

If you know the company you want to work for, go directly to the source. Employers often list specific jobs on their own Web sites, as do universities, departments of health, and other government agencies. The latter types of listings will often offer informative details on job descriptions, education and experience requirements, and salary ranges. Browsing a variety of sources will give you an idea of the job opportunities out there for an entry-level RD.

Job Bank Web Sites

- **CareerBuilder** (www.careerbuilder.com)
- **Idealist.org** (www.idealist.org)
- **iHireNutrition** (www.ihirenutrition.com)
- **Indeed** (www.indeed.com)
- **Monster** (www.monster.com)
- **Nutrition Jobs** (www.nutritionjobs.com)

Don't be discouraged if you see a listing for your dream job but it requires much more experience than you have right now. In fact, you should get excited that your dream job is out there and that someone has already outlined the roadmap of skills and experience you should work toward gaining to be a great candidate in the future. In the meantime, look for entry-level work that will help build the skills you need for the next step in your career.

Tools for the Job Hunt

Your tangible tools for the job hunt are your resume, cover letter, and marketing materials. You should also secure permission from three to four references to have their names and contact information provided to prospective employers.

For More Information

For additional guidance on putting together a resume, check out our other book, *Creating Your Career Portfolio: At-a-Glance Guide for Dietitians* (Prentice Hall, 2004). This book even takes it a step further by teaching food and nutrition professionals how to build career portfolios. This easy-to-read guidebook provides future RDs with the detailed instructions for planning, assembling, and using a career portfolio for career search or advancement. This text prepares students for the requirements of the American Dietetic Association, and it introduces them to the importance of pulling together all their qualifications, accomplishments, work samples, skills, and abilities to package them into a complete personalized portfolio.

The Resume

First of all, do you have a resume? There's no time like now to build one. Plan ahead so you do not find yourself needing one before it's created. If you have access to a university career center, it usually provides resume review services and can help you craft a strong resume.

Your internship director is another resource, as are many of the job bank Web sites listed in this chapter.

The Cover Letter

Your cover letter is a chance to show your potential employer that you are an effective and professional communicator. Our tips for how to write a great cover letter are similar to our tips for a winning resume: keep it short, professional, and tailor it to each job opportunity.

Your Marketing Materials

On marketing yourselves: we advise you to at minimum get business cards and stationery, and both must present you and your services in a professional manner. No tap-dancing broccoli or carrot sticks with shades! Create a positive image in all that you do, especially when it comes to having your name in print. There are even great design-it-yourself Web sites (which we both use), such as Vistaprint (www.vistaprint.com) and Overnight Prints (www.overnightprints.com).

Work Samples

You may consider putting together a packet of your past work that is most relevant to the job at hand. For example, if you're applying for a position in a community health center and part of the job description says you'd be creating educational materials, then you can provide copies of past educational handouts you've made and lesson plans. If the job is media spokesperson, maybe you provide a reel of morning shows you've been on. If you're applying for a position in a health advocacy office, you can show them copies of congressional testimony you've prepared in the past or a press release from a grassroots event you helped organize. The idea is to show that you have the experience to succeed and add value to their organization.

The Interview

When you've been invited for an interview, you're in a good place. It shows that your resume and cover letter were impressive enough to a prospective employer that they're interested in learning more about you to see if you truly will be a good fit for their organization. Thanks to the job research you've done, chances are you will be.

> ### Accounting for Gaps in Time
>
> If your resume contains gaps in time, be prepared to explain why those gaps occurred. Employers may ask. Perhaps you took time off to raise a family, further your education, or had a personal problem. Try to keep it positive, and avoid telling potential employers about health problems or sharing personal information that may expose unnecessary information.

The Salary Negotiation

Many people consider the salary negotiation to be their least favorite part of the process. We hope to provide useful tips for ensuring fair compensation and not selling yourself short. Remember that you have valuable, specialized skills and should be fairly compensated. In fact, not demanding fair compensation hurts the profession as a whole. That said, because the number of zeros on your paycheck is also a reflection of how you fit into an employer's overall budget, it's important to remember that our personal value is different than the concrete number of dollars we take home. For example, two smart, capable, entry-level RDs may find themselves taking home very different paychecks, with different benefits and vacation time, because one is leading a public school wellness program and the other works in a corporate public relations office. What we're trying to say is that the salary negotiation is about getting competitive compensation package for the type of job you're doing, in the field you're doing it in, rather than an actual number of dollars, vacation days, or benefits.

What's the Going Rate?

You've found a job you're interested in, now find the going rate for that type of position in your area. Perform your own informal surveys by asking your friends and colleagues about salaries. It may be more tactful to ask them about a range for the typical candidate who works in their city or their specific area or field. Also check government guides, like the Bureau of Labor Statistics' *Occupational Outlook Handbook*, and the American Dietetic Association's salary survey; also, many government positions will be upfront with salary ranges right in the job listing. Check out these Web sites to get started: Bureau of Labor Statistics (www.bls.gov), Riley Guide (www.rileyguide .com), and Salary.com (www.salary.com).

Be Bold

If you do not ask, you probably won't get—or at least that's what successful negotiators like to say. Dietetics isn't typically considered an extremely high-paying profession. It's also thought of as a women's profession, which is unsurprising as most RDs are female. Unfortunately, in the United States women tend to earn less than men. This isn't right, but it is true, and we should work to address the imbalance. We encourage you to engage in healthy negotiations with employers.

In your negotiations, wait to talk money until after the company or employer mentions it to you. Do not be the first to bring it up. Usually salary comes up after an offer is extended. When this happens,

> ### *Case Study in Salary Negotiations*
>
> Consuela was offered $45,000 to be clinical nutrition manager in a small urban hospital. She wanted $47,300, an amount equal to a 10 percent raise from her salary. She took two days to think about the offer and then called the hiring manager. She expressed her thanks for the offer but reiterated that she was looking for something closer to $47,000. The hiring manager said he could not meet that, so Consuela declined the job offer. One week later the recruiter called back and offered Consuela the 10 percent increase. As it turns out, it was a fair amount to ask for, and Consuela was the top candidate. She had done homework and was positioned to ask for what her performance was worth. Taking the risk paid off.

you want the employer to mention a figure first. Let them make you an offer so you know their position.

Staying Current

Did you know to stay current in this field you must read every single research article and abstract ever published? Well, actually, that's not true. Sorry to have alarmed you! However, once you're in the workforce, you may not have as much access to the colleagues that you used to see regularly in class and in internship rotations. For the working RD, staying current and connected does take some work, but we have tips and strategies to make it easier for you!

One thing you should do is subscribe to the American Dietetic Association's Knowledge Center *Daily News* (it's free). Each weekday morning, you will receive an e-mail with the most current headlines influencing the profession, and on Friday it includes a roundup of the top research findings for the week.

You can also read abstracts of research from other journals published in the back of the *Journal of the American Dietetic Association* and in the quarterly publication of the Dietitians in Nutrition Support dietetic practice group. As there's very little possibility that you can possibly read every study, it's more realistic to hit the high points by scanning these updates.

You should consider joining professional Listservs, such as those provided by dietetic practice groups you've joined. Staying connected and keeping up with colleagues will also help you keep up with what's going on in the professional world of food and nutrition.

These are just some of the ways to stay current. In the following resource lists, we identify some of the top sources of nutrition information to get you started, but these lists are by no means exhaustive.

Printed Newsletters and Magazines

The following printed periodicals require subscriptions:

- *Environmental Nutrition* (www.environmentalnutrition.com)
- *Nutrition Action Health Letter* (www.cspinet.org/nah)
- *Tufts University Health & Nutrition Letter* (www.tuftshealthletter.com)
- *The Johns Hopkins Medical Letter: Health After 50* (www.hopkinsafter50.com)
- Harvard Health Letters (www.health.harvard.edu):
  - *Harvard Women's Health Watch*
  - *Harvard Men's Health Watch*
  - *Harvard Heart Letter*
- *Berkeley's Wellness Letter* (www.berkeleywellness.com)
- *Today's Dietitian* (www.todaysdietitian.com)

Nutrition Publications Available Only to ADA Members

For subscription and access information for the following ADA members-only publications, go to the Member Center on the ADA Web site (www.eatright.org/Member):

- *Journal of the American Dietetic Association:* The premier source for the practice and science of food, nutrition, and dietetics.
- *ADA Student Scoop*: The online newsletter exclusively for dietetics students.
- *ADA Times*: Quarterly magazine that gives you the latest trends and opportunities in the dietetics profession in addition to research briefs and industry trends, hot topics in nutrition, professional development resources, public policy issues, and Association news.
- *Behind the Scenes at ADA*: Connects first-year active members with ADA benefits and services.
- *CADE Connection*: Accreditation decisions and updates.
- *Daily News:* The latest news on food, nutrition, and health
- *Eat Right Weekly:* Weekly Web-based newsletter includes On the Pulse of Public Policy, CPE Corner, Career Resources, Research Briefs, ADA Member Updates, Philanthropy, Awards, and Grants.
- *MNT Provider:* Monthly newsletter that helps explain the complexities of Medicare and other reimbursement issues.

Online Publications

Current and back issues of the following publications are available on the Internet:

- Kansas State University Nutrition Extension *Nutrition News* (http://www.ksre.ksu.edu/humannutrition; select Newsletters from Home page menu)
- U.S. Department of Agriculture (USDA) *Nutrition Insights* (www.cnpp.usda.gov/nutritioninsights.htm)
- USDA *Nutrition and Your Child* (www.kidsnutrition.org)
- *National Food Service Management Institute's NFSMI Insight* (www.nfsmi.org)
- *MCH (Maternal and Child Health) Research to Practice* (www.ncemch.org/research/diss.html#1)
- *University of Nebraska–Lincoln Food Reflections Newsletter* (http://lancaster.unl.edu/food/food-reflections.shtml)
- USDA Agriculture Research Service *Food and Nutrition Research Briefs* (www.ars.usda.gov/is/np/fnrb)
- *Feeding Kids Newsletter* (www.nutritionforkids.com)
- University of Texas Southwestern Medical Center *Center for Human Nutrition Newsletter* (www.utsouthwestern.edu; to access newsletter, search "Center for Human Nutrition")
- *American Institute for Cancer Research Newsletter* (www.aicr.org/publications)
- *Foodsafe.* www.foodsafety.gov/news/educators

Some of the "Big" Journals

The following is a list of high-quality peer-reviewed academic journals in which nutrition-related research articles may appear:

- *American Journal of Clinical Nutrition*
- *American Journal of Public Health*
- *Archives of Internal Medicine*
- *British Medical Journal*
- *Cambridge Scientific Abstracts*

- *Circulation*
- *Diabetes*
- *Diabetes/Metabolism Research and Reviews*
- *Family Economics and Nutrition Review*
- *International Journal of Eating Disorders*
- *International Journal of Obesity*
- *Journal of the American College of Nutrition*
- *Journal of the American Dietetic Association*
- *Journal of the American Medical Association (JAMA)*
- *Medical Student JAMA*
- *Journal of Nutrition*
- *Journal of Nutrition Education and Behavior*
- *Journal of Parenteral and Enteral Nutrition*
- *New England Journal of Medicine*
- *Nutrition in Clinical Practice*
- *Nutrition: International Journal of Applied and Basic Nutritional Sciences*
- *Obesity Research*

A Closer Look

Polishing Your Image: How to Become Socially Savvy In Business Relations

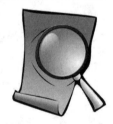

By Lisa Mosing, MS, RD, FADA, President, NutriTalk, Inc.

Image speaks volumes about our business. Our clients are constantly confronted with poised and polished media-savvy professionals giving advice or pitching a product. No matter how much technical or nutritional expertise you possess, a polished image can help make the deal. Unfortunately, in to-day's society, it is often not just what you know but how you present your skills and experiences.

1. **Make a lasting impression in person and on paper.** In person you can let your voice, posture, and body language convey your enthusiasm and interest. We all know to sit attentively, watch the face of the other person talking, and listen to what they are saying. But take a look at your paper image as well. Does it match your persona? Does it command attention? Is it professional? Cohesive written materials that are professional and reflect your personal style take time to produce. Part of a paper image is a business name and logo. You may want to consider the implication of registering your name and logo, as this is an important consideration in designing your business as an asset. Remember that all written communications are permanent and used as reference to your business and your image.

2. **Communication is vital.** It can't be said enough how important communication is to image. Take a look at how you communicate, and then look at your clients, potential clients, and competitors. Listen to your language, word choice, and tone when you answer the phone or meet with a client. Do you speak their language or use a lot of lingo or technical terms? Would your client prefer to have written information to refer to and "digest" before or after the meeting? Identify the preferred communication mode for your clients and use it. Break down how you send your message to potential clients—is there a better way to get their attention?

3. **Use the introduction to your advantage.** Imagine yourself as you are introduced. What impression do you make?

Plan a confident introduction. Practice a 10-second "commercial" for your introduction. Everyone, at one point or another, forgets a name when they try to introduce people. A person will not be upset if you are honest. Most experts agree that it is best to admit your lapse in memory. Then say something you remember about the person whose name you cannot recall. If you are on the receiving end of someone who has forgotten your name, do not make them suffer. Put out your hand, state your name, and greet them. The response will be relief.

4. **Don't let down time take down your image.** A good business professional keeps to their schedule and considers the feelings of their clients and coworkers when there are interruptions and delays. If you must keep someone waiting, greet them, apologize for your delay, and let them know how long you will be delayed. When you have down time while waiting for a client or when visiting another business, use it to your advantage to update your planner or organize your thoughts. But remember that cell phones may not always be welcome. Turn your phone off before your meeting, or better yet, you may want to leave it in the car.

5. **Final thoughts.** Well-educated professionals often sabotage their efforts by neglecting the common courtesy of a thank-you note. You need to stand out as a professional in the competitive marketplace. An articulate, persuasive, and carefully composed letter will polish your professional image and can add to your success. Letters of acknowledgement and thanks are also an important part of executive communications. It is not enough to call, e-mail, or fax a thank you, unless that is the preferred method of communication. Otherwise, a handwritten note is appreciated and is often more effective. The

Nutrition Entrepreneurs dietetic practice group is a great place to hone your business skills. We have various resources in the NE lending library, experts in our NE membership, and advice available from the NE Listserv to help make you a more poised and polished nutrition expert. Good luck!

Reprinted from Ventures, *Spring 2003. Used by permission of the author.* *http://nutritalk.com.*

7

Movers and Shakers

In this book, we have focused on showing you dietetics inside and out. We illustrate what it takes to succeed in school, how to conquer the dietetic internship application and land an internship, where to go for volunteer experiences, and so much more. Now we offer you profiles of several key individuals we deem movers and shakers in the field of food and nutrition. These folks know how to work well with others, build influential alliances, and function as savvy businesspeople. They are true trailblazers, taking their careers to the maximum by doing all the things we've described in this text. (In fact, many will have moved on to new adventures and accomplishments by the time these profiles are published!) Read on as each shares his or her career aspirations, accomplishments, and words of wisdom.

Clinical Management:
Pam Charney, PhD, RD

Biography

Pam Charney, PhD, RD, completed her undergraduate studies at the University of West Florida and was a dietetic intern at Walter Reed Army Medical Center. She went on to earn her PhD at the University of Medicine and Dentistry of New Jersey.

> ### Pam Charney's Current Passion
>
> To develop tools for RDs who require rapid access to information in practice.

Pam is currently a faculty member and master's student at the University of Washington, where she studies clinical informatics. She hopes to develop informatics competencies for RDs and ensure representation of dietetics in the electronic health record.

Pam's previous experience includes being a nutrition support dietitian, pediatric dietitian, and clinical nutrition manager at Madigan Army Medical Center, as well as more than 20 years' experience as a practitioner and manager in a variety of settings, from small community hospitals to large teaching hospitals.

Pam and her husband Dave are the parents of three daughters.

AWARDS AND HONORS

Pam was the first dietitian selected to receive a National Library of Medicine fellowship to attend the Biomedical Informatics Short Course at Woods Hole, and she was invited to the 2006 Nursing Informatics TIGER meeting. Her other awards and honors include:

- American Dietetic Association (ADA) Award for Excellence in Clinical Nutrition

- Dietitians in Nutrition Support (DNS) Distinguished Nutrition Support Dietitian Award
- American Society for Parenteral and Enteral Nutrition (ASPEN) Outstanding Nutrition Support Dietitian Award
- ADA Foundation Medallion Award
- Outstanding Alumna by the University of Medicine and Dentistry of New Jersey (2006)

GIVING BACK TO THE PROFESSION

Pam's contributions to the dietetics community are extensive. For example, she has served as:

- Director, ADA House of Delegates
- Member, ADA Board of Directors
- Charter member, ADA Standardized Language Committee
- Member, ADA Research Committee
- Web site manager, DNS dietetic practice group (DPG)
- Past chair, DNS DPG
- ASPEN Board of Directors

Career Reflections

"I have loved every moment of my career, although some of those moments have been loved in hindsight. I was fortunate to be mentored, both formally and informally, by many outstanding clinicians. I sought role models from all areas of health care, not just dietetics. I think this gave me the broad perspective needed for effective practice. Reaching out to others also helped me solidify my role as the nutrition expert on the health care team because my colleagues from other areas were familiar with my knowledge and expertise.

"While I've held a variety of positions throughout my career, I think my favorites were working in critical care and working with children who have short gut syndrome. Both populations are very complex and require a nimble mind to adjust care plans frequently and often with little additional information. Providing nutrition care to these fragile patients also required that I reach out to other clinicians to ensure that everyone's goals were considered.

"I recently received a thank-you note from one of our program graduates. Her note said 'thanks for standing up for me and our profession.' I think this spoke volumes; it's easy to become defensive and hide in one's office when others behave with more assertiveness than we're comfortable with. I make it a point to teach students that if you've chosen this career, then you have to take the responsibility to stand up for your career choice. To do so you have to not only possess a certain level of assertiveness but you also have to 'know your stuff.'

> ## Pam Charney's Words of Wisdom
>
> - Decide where you want to be in the future and take the steps to begin on that path.
> - Having a firm goal in mind helps direct many of the choices that we have to make in life.

"I love knowing that the nutrition care I provided made it possible for patients to survive critical illness. I've seen the joy on the faces of children with short gut who learn how to savor the experience of eating."

Communications: Liz Marr, MS, RD

Biography

Liz Marr, MS, RD, principal and founder, Liz Marr and Associates, LLC, in Longmont, Colorado, is a food and nutrition communications expert with 20 years of experience in the field, specializing in health, food, nutrition, textile arts, and agriculture. A veteran writer and spokesperson, she has participated in nearly 1,000 media interviews.

Liz received a master of science degree in food and nutrition science from Colorado State University, and she graduated cum laude from University of Missouri, Columbia, with a bachelor of science degree in family and consumer sciences, specializing in fashion merchandising.

Steps in Liz's career have included the following:

> ## Liz Marr's Current Passion
>
> To continue building my food and nutrition communications career, be a role model for other food and nutrition professionals, and balance my professional with my personal life.

- Cofounder of Marr Barr Communications in Longmont, a women- and RD-owned public relations firm specializing in food, nutrition, and agriculture, including natural and organic products
- Manager of consumer communications for Horizon Organic Dairy, in Boulder, Colorado
- Vice president of programs for the Western Dairy Council and Western Dairyfarmers' Promotion Association, in Thornton, Colorado

AWARDS AND HONORS

Liz has been honored with the following:

- Colorado Dietetic Association's Outstanding Dietitian of the Year (2004)
- Colorado Young Dietitian of the Year Award

GIVING BACK TO THE PROFESSION

Among her many accomplishments, Liz has served the food and nutrition profession as:

- Chair, Food and Culinary Professionals DPG
- Society for Nutrition Education Foundation Board of Trustees
- Chair, Nutrition and Food Science Section of the International Association of Culinary Professionals
- President, Colorado Dietetic Association
- Chair, Nutrition Education for the Public DPG
- ADA spokesperson
- Board, Boulder County Safehouse (now Safehouse Progressive Alliance for Nonviolence) in Boulder, Colorado

Career Reflections

"I was a junior in college majoring in fashion merchandising when I received a call from my mom that my father was scheduled for a triple bypass because he had had a mild heart attack. Now enjoying a healthy lifestyle in his 70s, my dad was only 47 at the time. He had gone in for a checkup because his twin brother had been diagnosed with coronary artery blockage requiring bypass surgery.

"That experience led me to take a nutrition class as an elective my senior year. It was then that I realized I wanted a career in dietetics. Over the years, I have had the good fortune to have the support of numerous mentors in the field, and it was my boss in the Migrant Health program, the Colorado Dietetic Association president at the time, who referred me to the local Dairy Council, where I started my first full-time position after graduate school. One of the reasons I was

Liz Marr's Words of Wisdom

- Make friends, ask questions, strive for high-quality performance, set your boundaries, and charge what you are worth.
- What goes around comes around: Volunteer and nurture those around you—you will gain far more than you give.

hired was my experience and education in communications and marketing. I stayed with the Dairy Council for 12 years.

"Amy Barr and I cofounded Marr Barr Communications in 2000 after working together at Horizon Organic Dairy, and we enjoyed a successful eight-year run as a strategic marketing and communications agency specializing in food, nutrition, health, lifestyle, and sustainability, with five full-time team members and a prestigious client list. I currently enjoy a high degree of independence with my current consulting practice, working from home, actively engaging in social media, teaching part-time at Front Range Community College, and enjoying volunteer experiences. The choice to be self-employed has allowed me the flexibility to balance my personal and professional endeavors and has been immensely rewarding."

Community Nutrition: Jo Ann Millsap Pegues, MPA, RD

Biography

Jo Ann Millsap Pegues is the project manager for Focus on Diabetes at the Center for African American Health in Denver, Colorado. Her additional training includes a certificate in adult weight management through the ADA and Commission on Dietetic Registration (CDR) (2001) and a one-year fellowship with the Regional Institute for Health and Environmental Leadership at the University of Denver and the University of Colorado Health Sciences Center. Other highlights of her career history include working as a program

> **Jo Ann Millsap Pegues's Current Passion**
>
> To work in the community promoting good nutrition and physical activity to African Americans and provide private consultation to persons needing individualized services.

specialist at the U.S. Administration on Aging and serving as acting regional program director, team leader, state liaison, and chief of program development for the Administration on Aging.

AWARDS AND HONORS

Among the accolades Jo Ann has received are the following:

- Distinguished alumni from the School of Health and Environmental Science at Oklahoma State University (2003)
- ADA Medallion Award (2001)

GIVING BACK TO THE PROFESSION

Jo Ann is past president and treasurer of the Colorado Dietetic Association and has held several elected and appointed positions in ADA, including two terms on ADA's Diversity Committee, and as president of the National Organization of Blacks in Nutrition and Dietetics, for which she was elected to the nominating committee for the 2010–2011 term.

Career Reflections

"As a student at Oklahoma State University, I had a wonderful adviser who was genuinely interested in me—one of less than 30 African American students in the entire university—and my success. She advised me upon graduation to become a member of ADA, become involved, and never let my membership drop. I have appreciated her advice and followed it throughout my career.

"When I moved from Oklahoma to Denver, I became involved in the Denver Dietetic Association and volunteered for various committees, where I met dietitians who encouraged and supported me, and they became lifelong friends.

"This was the beginning of my volunteerism in the profession that has resulted in my involvement not only at the district and state levels, but also in several elected positions in ADA. In 2001, I was recognized with the Medallion Award, which was a career highlight.

"A willingness to volunteer your time makes a difference both on the job and professionally. Once your name is familiar, other opportunities arise. I was willing to say yes because there were so few African Americans in the profession, and what I learned over the years was that you often have to do more than others just to be recognized for your knowledge, skills, and abilities.

"Now my goals are to do the very best I can in my current position and share my nutrition knowledge with others along the way. My parents taught me to do my best in any situation, which I have tried to do, and with the support and encouragement of my husband and family, it's been a pleasant journey. I know that in the Book of Life, we are not responsible for the beginning or the end, but for the chapters in between. I have tried to make those chapters interesting, helpful, encouraging, fun, and unforgettable."

Jo Ann Millsap Pegues's Words of Wisdom

- Choosing a career in nutrition requires commitment and hard work.
- It is a most rewarding career, but it is up to the individual to make the most of it.

Critical Care:
Marion F. Winkler, PhD, RD, CNSC

Biography

Marion F. Winkler, PhD, RD, CNSC, is the surgical nutrition specialist at Rhode Island Hospital. With over 25 years' experience in nutrition support practice, Marion is also associate professor of surgery in the Alpert Medical School of Brown University. Marion has published numerous articles and chapters on nutrition assessment, parenteral nutrition, quality assurance in nutrition support practice, and quality of life of home parenteral nutrition patients. Reflecting on her career highlights, she notes, "I have had the opportunity to coordinate a nutrition course for second-year medical students at Brown University and currently contribute lectures in nutrition assessment and nutritional support as well as precept dietetic interns and medical students during clinical rotations. I also play a significant role in the training of surgical residents and fellows in gastroenterology and critical care."

Marion earned her bachelor of science in nutrition from Case Western Reserve University, in Cleveland, Ohio; her master of science in allied health from the University of Connecticut; and PhD in health sciences from the University of Medicine and Dentistry of New Jersey. She resides in Cranston, Rhode Island, with her husband Larry and two daughters.

> ## Marion Winkler's Five-Year Goal
>
> Develop and validate a patient-reported outcomes questionnaire to assess quality of life for home parenteral nutrition–dependent individuals, and enhance my nutrition curricula.

Awards and Honors

Marion's awards and honors include:

- ADA Medallion Award
- Lenna Frances Cooper Lecture at FNCE (2009)
- Distinguished Award in Nutrition Support Dietetics

Giving Back to the Profession

Marion's contributions to the food and nutrition profession are demonstrated by the following accomplishments:

- Chair, ADA's Dietitians in Nutrition Support DPG
- Delegate from Rhode Island, ADA House of Delegates

- Council on Professional Issues Delegate for Clinical Nutrition, ADA House of Delegates
- First dietitian to serve as president of ASPEN
- Board of Directors, ASPEN Rhoads Research Foundation
- Board of Trustees, Oley Foundation

Career Reflections

"Caring for critically ill patients has been one of the most challenging aspects of my job, but knowing I have played a part in their recovery is also extremely rewarding. These patients have extraordinarily high energy and nutrient requirements because of the magnitude of their injuries and lengthy hospitalization and rehabilitation. I have established close relationships with many of my patients, and as a result I am committed to finding ways to improve their quality of life.

"I draw from my clinical experiences to support the academic teaching that I do. What has made me an effective teacher is remaining involved in clinical practice. I am able to give students examples of real patients from my own experience. I think this makes a tremendous and long-lasting impression. In recognition of these accomplishments, my department has supported my pending promotion to associate professor of surgery.

"I am indebted to the terrific role models I had as an undergraduate and graduate student. The nutrition and dietetics faculty at Case Western Reserve University, the University of Connecticut, and the University of Medicine and Dentistry of New Jersey were enthusiastic, motivating, and challenging. Not only did I gain knowledge and practical experience, I was exposed and encouraged to participate in our professional association activities. Having now attended three

Marion Winkler's Words of Wisdom

- Work hard and remain challenged.
- Find good role models and mentor others.

universities that were homes to former ADA presidents, it is not surprising that I have followed in their leadership footsteps! Professional volunteerism has become a way of life for me.

"One of the greatest rewards and benefits of sustaining a career in nutrition support dietetics has been the friends I have made. My professional colleagues have become my closest friends. I feel constantly motivated by these individuals and challenged to contribute as much as possible to better the profession."

Culinary Nutrition: Jackie Newgent, RD

Biography

Jackie Newgent is a dietitian-chef, cookbook author, culinary instructor, freelance writer, media spokesperson, and culinary and nutrition communications consultant in New York, New York. Recently, she authored *Big Green Cookbook* (Wiley, 2009) and the award-winning *The All-Natural Diabetes Cookbook* (American Diabetes Association, 2007). Jackie appears frequently as a health, eco-cuisine, and culinary nutrition expert on television and radio, and she is the "In Season" columnist for *Edible Queens* and advisory board member for *Fitness*. She's also a past national media spokesperson for ADA.

> ### Jackie Newgent's Current Passion
>
> Have two more cookbooks published and be a sidekick or star of a television or Web-based food show.

Jackie received her bachelor of science in allied health professions from the Ohio State University and her certificate in professional cooking from Kendall College. In her career, she has worked as a staff nutritionist in Ohio working with obesity, consulted at rehabilitation centers and long-term care facilities, and been involved in nutrition education program planning and corporate health promotion. She has served as a nutrition educator at the Culinary School of Kendall College and instructor at the Institute of Culinary Education. Jackie's Web site is jackienewgent.com.

GIVING BACK TO THE PROFESSION

In addition to serving as an ADA national media spokesperson, Jackie has supported the food and nutrition profession as an ADA Consumer Nutrition Hotline dietitian, and she is an active member of the Food and Culinary Professionals dietetic practice group.

Career Reflections

"My first word wasn't 'mommy' or 'daddy' but an Arabic word for food. My mother, a caterer, taught me to love food. Together with my mom, we would carefully inspect sides of naturally raised beef, only purchase fresh chicken coming from a trusted nearby local farm, and seasonally pluck fresh wild grape leaves from nearby vines for my favorite childhood dish, stuffed grape leaves. It was these early life lessons rooted in good food that have been some of the most important in shaping my career. My passion for food has stuck with me all of my life.

> ### Jackie Newgent's Words of Wisdom
>
> - Keep following your dream—even when you hit a couple "nightmares" along your journey.
> - Create your own career niche if it doesn't already exist.

"While working in Chicago, I was interviewed on national TV a few times. That gave me a 'bug' for media work. After hundreds of print, radio, and television interviews and numerous media contacts, I launched my career as a culinary nutritionist specializing in communications. Now, I'm a food industry spokesperson, speak professionally at national conferences, and regularly contribute recipes and menus to national magazines. And I'm thrilled to say that I also have two published cookbooks. The more I'm read, heard, or seen, the more opportunities arise. In other words, marketing made easy.

"Another self-marketing key is my involvement with professional membership groups and associations, such as the Food and Culinary Professionals DPG. I was on their board for several years—and wholeheartedly enjoyed the experience. I feel so lucky to have a career that's happily intertwined with my life."

Dietetics Leadership/Strategic Planning: Marianne Smith Edge, MS, RD, FADA

Biography

Since 1986, Marianne Smith Edge, MS, RD, FADA, has been owner and president of MSE & Associates, LLC, a nutrition communications and strategic planning consulting firm in Owensboro, Kentucky. Her expertise includes health and wellness and sustainability issues, farm-to-table policy issues, strategic positioning of nutritional products and services, development of workshops and seminars, writing for professional audiences, and as a nationally recognized speaker. Having been raised on a dairy farm and a partner in two family farms, Marianne understands the agricultural sustainability issues from producer to consumer.

> **Marianne Smith Edge's Current Passion**
>
> National recognition for my company as a bridge between agriculture, food science, and nutrition to feed the world responsibly, and changing organizations through strategic planning.

Marianne holds a bachelor of science degree in dietetics from the University of Kentucky and a master's degree in public health-nutrition from Western Kentucky University. In her career, she has served on the USDA National Research, Extension, Education, and Economics Advisory Board; been a member of the University of Kentucky Board of Trustees; and worked as producer of a family and consumer science television program for the University of Kentucky College of Agriculture Extension Service.

AWARDS AND HONORS

Among the honors Marianne has received is the 2009 American Dietetic Association Medallion Award.

GIVING BACK TO THE PROFESSION

Marianne is a past president of the ADA and chaired the ADA Ethics Committee.

Career Reflections

"Since becoming a registered dietitian 28 years ago, building a career in dietetics and involvement in the American Dietetic Association have been synonymous. It was the encouragement and opportunities afforded by my boss and peers at my first job, working for a long-term care corporation, that opened the door for involvement with the Kentucky Dietetic Association and the Consultant Dietitians in Healthcare Facilities (CD-HCF) dietetic practice group (now called Dietetics in Health Care Communities).

"At one point, when I lost my job, I was happy to have a support network of consultant dietitians through CD-HCF. These women, serving as wonderful mentors, fueled my dream to start a consulting business. My first contract with a health care product manufacturer was originally initiated due to my involvement with ADA. Success in any area of dietetics requires commitment and the understanding that there will always be peaks and valleys along the way.

"Over the years, I have learned that establishing a viable business requires networking, staying on the cutting edge of your area of expertise, and understanding that dietetics is a business. Throughout my career, connecting with colleagues has led to career advancement, collaboration on books and magazine articles, as well as developing a wealth of knowledge that has enhanced my career and personal growth.

"My involvement with CD-HCF truly was the springboard to my long-standing commitment to the profession and ADA. Professional growth opportunities within practice groups to the House of Delegates and association-wide committees provided the foundation for my involvement with the ADA Board of Directors as director-at-large, House of Delegate speaker, and president.

"Each of these roles has provided me invaluable experience with strategic planning, knowledge-based strategic governance, association management, board facilitation, and member development. The knowledge and leadership skills I have gained are priceless!"

Marianne Smith Edge's Words of Wisdom

- Leadership is about giving of yourself to make an organization, profession, or your personal life better for all.
- It's about doing the right thing.

Disordered Eating: Jessica Setnick, MS, RD

Jessica Setnick's Current Passion

Keep doing what I'm doing to reach a broader and wider audience in order to better prevent and treat disordered eating.

Biography

A private practitioner in Dallas, Texas, Jessica Setnick, MS, RD, CSSD, is the founder of "Eating Disorders Boot Camp" and author of the *ADA Pocket Guide to Eating Disorders* (2011). She is best known for her straightforward approach to treating eating disorders and educating the public and other health professionals. As the owner of UnderstandingNutrition.com and EatingDisorderJobs.com, Jessica provides what professionals in the eating disorders field need most: confidence, competence, and community. Knowing that many of us work in isolated settings, Jessica is always looking for ways to use new technology to bring us together with the ultimate goal of improving dietetics education to include more about eating disorders.

Career Reflections

"Being a dietitian has been incredibly rewarding and at times very trying. I have found that many people have a limited or incorrect view of dietitians, even in the eating disorders field. There are so many possibilities of careers, projects, and options once you have the degrees and qualifications. There is no limit, but there is also not always a path. I have been very entrepreneurial, but there are times when I wish that I just had 'one job' with someone to tell me what to do. These moments are usually short-lived, because I remember that when I had a boss, I never liked being told what to do or how to do it. Being 'successfully unemployed,' as I call it, for almost 10 years now has taught me a lot about the world, myself, and how I relate to others.

"I have grown up a lot having to make my own decisions, because in private practice there is no one to blame when things go wrong. It has been a long and winding road, but I wouldn't have it any other way. I have had opportunities to travel, impact the lives of students, and participate in

Jessica Setnick's Words of Wisdom

- If you know what you want to accomplish, ask people for advice that can get you there, not for their opinions on whether you should proceed.

- If you are committed to your idea, you don't need anyone else's approval to go for it or anyone else's doubts to rain on your parade.

the business world and the media in ways that I don't believe would have been open to me had I stayed in the clinical setting. I have learned to have goals but to also be open to the opportunities that arise along the path—they sometimes take me to new goals that I wasn't even aware of.

"My nutrition education, even with my master's degree, was only the basis for what I do now. Everything since then I have learned through continuing education, seeking out advisers, and reading up on the topics I need. Most of the time I feel incredibly lucky and happy to be able to come in to my office every day and do what I do."

Extended Care/Assisted Living Nutrition: Becky Dorner, RD

Biography

Widely known as one of the nation's leading experts on nutrition and long-term care issues, Becky Dorner, RD, has more than 25 years' experience as a speaker, consultant, and author. She is president of Becky Dorner & Associates, Inc., in Akron, Ohio, which publishes and presents continuing education programs and information on nutrition care for older adults and other topics; and Becky Dorner & Associates Consulting, which since 1983 has employed RDs and DTRs to provide services to health care facilities in Ohio and western Pennsylvania. Becky's mission to improve care for older adults has inspired her to present more than 500 programs for national, international, and state professional meetings

Becky Dorner's Current Passion

Increase how many people we reach through consulting, publications, and educational events, and develop a succession plan to keep the company thriving into the future.

in 5 countries and 48 states and to publish more than 220 manuals, continuing education programs, and practical articles for professional journals and newsletters. Her previous work experience included conducting one-on-one counseling and group classes and being a foodservice dietitian.

GIVING BACK TO THE PROFESSION

Becky's contributions to the field of dietetics include:

- Chair, Dietetics in Health Care Communities
- Delegate, ADA House of Delegates
- Board officer, National Pressure Ulcer Advisory Panel
- Member, ADA Research Committee
- Member, ADA Evidence Analysis Unintentional Weight Loss Work Group

HONORS AND AWARDS

Becky's notable achievements include the following:

- ADA Award of Excellence in Business and Consultation
- DHCC Distinguished Member Award
- Nutrition Entrepreneurs DPG Outstanding Nutrition Entrepreneur
- ADA Recognized Young Dietitian of the Year

Career Reflections

"I love being in dietetics—the opportunities are endless! I have had the wonderful opportunity to experience life as an entrepreneur and business owner since 1983. I always knew I wanted to be an entrepreneur. Within two years of college graduation and with absolutely no money to back me, I started Becky Dorner & Associates Consulting. I really knew nothing about being in business, but I had an inner drive that kept me moving forward no matter what the obstacles and challenges. At least I called it drive and perseverance—others would say I was crazy.

"Dietetics licensure had just passed in our state, and the need for RDs in long-term care was going to increase. For me, 'go where the market is' meant going to long-term care. Within six months of opening my consultant's business, I had more work than I could handle, and I brought on my first RD. Soon we had five full-time dietitians and nutrition associates on staff, and business kept growing from there.

Becky Dorner's Words of Wisdom

- Share your contacts, and bring people together to help each other.
- Learn how to have some balance to keep yourself and your family happy.

"As I grew my business, I stayed very involved with the dietetic association, serving in local, state, and then national positions with ADA. My volunteer work helped me to hone my speaking, writing, and leadership skills. As an added bonus, I have many wonderful friends from all over the country and abroad. I know the experts in each area of dietetics, so I can reach out for assistance any time I need it. I have a network of people that I refer others to, and I in turn receive referrals. My network expanded outside the field of dietetics as I have networked with many other entrepreneurs over the years, and also with many other professionals in complementary industries.

"All of this has helped me to grow a profitable business that has enriched my life and achieved our mission of improving the lives of older adults through excellent nutrition care. And best of all, it has supported my family of five and the families of more than twenty other fabulous professionals in our company."

Foodservice Management/Education:
Linda J. Lafferty, PhD, RD, FADA

Biography

Linda is director of the dietetic internship, associate director of food and nutrition services, and associate professor at Rush University Medical Center in Chicago. She is a past president of the American Society for Healthcare Foodservice Management, and she continues to serve as chair of the education team. In addition, she has also held elected positions in the Foodservice Systems Management Education Council and other professional associations.

> **Linda Lafferty's Current Passion**
>
> Positively touch the future of dietetics practice through my students.

A native of Fayetteville, Arkansas, Linda worked as a medical dietitian at the University of Arkansas Medical Center and Baptist Memorial Hospital in Little Rock before earning a PhD in food systems management from the University of Missouri, Columbia. She has published, received many awards, and been invited as a featured speaker. She has also previously served on the faculty at Louisiana State University, Baton Rouge, and the University of Tennessee, Knoxville, and worked as director of food and nutrition services at Rush University Medical Center.

Awards and Honors

Linda is a Fellow, American Dietetic Association (FADA).

Giving Back to the Profession

In addition to her service to the American Society for Healthcare Foodservice Management (past president; current chair, education team) and Foodservice Systems Management Education Council (elected officer), Linda has been a member of the ADA Commission on Dietetic Registration and the Future Practice and Education Task Force, She has also been a program reviewer for the Commission on Accreditation for Dietetics Education and a member of the management workgroup.

Career Reflections

"My career in dietetics emerged from my desire to become a physician. Unfortunately, I was born about 20 years too soon for that goal to be realized. In 1967, my junior year of college, my premed adviser told me the medical school admissions committee would view my application as coming from a woman who would probably marry within her first two years of med school, drop out, and thus deprive some worthy young man of the opportunity to complete a medical education! Although this advice would be grounds for litigation today, in the 1960s, it was the way of life!

"Since my mom and older sister were dietitians, I had insight into the profession and enjoyed hearing their conversations about nutrition research. I decided to study nutrition and dietetics on my journey to medical school. As an RD member of the medical team, I learned that I didn't want to go to medical school, and I learned that I didn't want to be an RD member of the medical team!

"For me, the excitement and challenge of dietetics practice came from the management and administrative assignments I was given. However, my academic preparation in management was weak. Marion Spears, one of my undergraduate professors, had just completed her PhD under Aimee Moore at the University of Missouri, Columbia. She encouraged me to explore its foodservice systems management program. After a long weekend with students and faculty, I knew where I was going!

"Some of the most stimulating experiences in my doctoral program occurred in Aimee's home while she entertained visiting 'dignitaries' of the American Dietetic Association. I met more ADA presidents and leaders in Dr. Moore's dining room than at ADA conventions! I remember the first time I met Gertrude Blaker and Virginia Harger; I could barely resist asking for autographs!

"My first elected position in ADA was on the Commission on Dietetic Registration in 1982. I should have been charged tuition for that experience! The people with whom I had the honor to work were exceptional mentors and teachers. Since then, I have served ADA in some capacity on various councils and commissions related to dietetics practice, education, and credentialing."

Linda Lafferty's Words of Wisdom

- Life is a thrilling journey of educational opportunities taught by every person you meet and each place you visit along the way.
- Don't be afraid of taking the turns or exits along the way: the scenery and opportunities get more interesting the further you travel.

Nutrition Care in HIV/AIDS: Jennifer Muir Bowers, PhD, RD, CNSD

Biography

Currently, Jennifer teaches part-time for the University of Phoenix and Central Arizona College, works as a consultant on various writing and educational projects, and is a full-time mom to her daughter in Oro Valley, Arizona. Previously, she was a faculty member and adviser at the University of Arizona. She has more than 18 years of clinical nutrition experience, including time spent as a clinical dietitian at the Tucson VA Medical Center, and her work has appeared in peer-reviewed journals, books, and lay literature. She earned her PhD in nutritional sciences, with a minor in microbiology and immunology, from the University of Arizona. Her dietetic internship was completed at the Veterans Affairs Medical Center in Houston, Texas.

GIVING BACK TO THE PROFESSION

Jennifer has served in various leadership positions for the Infectious Diseases Nutrition (formerly HIV/AIDS) DPG.

AWARDS AND HONORS

Jennifer has received numerous awards and fellowships, including:

- Arizona Dietetic Association's Recognized Young Dietitian of the Year
- Emerging Leader Award, Arizona Dietetic Association
- E. Neige Todhunter Memorial Doctoral Fellowship
- Dietetic Educators of Practitioners Graduate Scholarship
- University of Arizona Food Science Fellowship
- A+ Adviser Award for the College of Agriculture and Life Sciences
- Outstanding Student Organization Adviser Award from the University of Arizona

Career Reflections

"I never meant to be a dietitian! My goal in life was to be a physician. I thought the money in a medical career would make me happy. I majored in nutrition in college but with medical school in mind. When I realized that working a million hours per week was not my idea of a high-quality lifestyle and that my clinical nutrition courses were invigorating, stimulating, and fun, I pursued dietetics.

"During my internship at the Houston VA Medical Center, I met the director and my mentor, Dr. Sydney Morrow. She was amazing— so smart, so challenging, so funny. I vowed to be just like her someday and work in dietetics education. During that internship, I found that I enjoyed critical care and teaching.

"Working in the intensive care units was rewarding as I figured out the intricate details of intravenous and tube feedings. Soon I was asked to participate in the HIV/AIDS team and began a mentoring relationship with Neil Ampel, MD, a highly respected and amazing physician. My interest in research began in Houston but really grew during my time with the HIV/AIDS team.

"The drive to conduct research is what landed me in the doctoral program at the University of Arizona. I was offered a faculty position, and as I had speculated back in Houston, I found that my true talents and passion were teaching in the classroom. I loved connecting with the students, planning lessons and lectures, seeing the light bulbs go off in their heads, and bringing my clinical experience to the classroom.

Jennifer Muir Bowers's Words of Wisdom

- Make the most of the situation you are in, because there is always something to learn and always room to grow.
- Never give up your dream, and never let anyone tell you that you can't!

"It is so true that everything that you experience in your life has a purpose. I had no idea that the spark that went off when I met Dr. Sydney Morrow would ignite into a full-blown passion for education. I never knew that working with Dr. Neil Ampel would lead to his directing my doctoral dissertation. I am not completely sure what my future holds, but I will continue to work in the areas that I have an enthusiasm for and see what unfolds before me."

Integrative Health: Jeff Fine, MS, MSW

Biography

In a career spanning two decades, Jeff's mission has been helping people find happiness and fulfillment by working with them to optimize their emotional and physical health. He has conducted thousands of sessions with individuals, families, and couples struggling with a broad array of mind-body conditions. These include conditions such as anxiety, depression, food- or weight-related issues, addiction, and relational problems. He has found that addressing the whole person (the "total self") is the most effective way to help clients make transformative changes that give them the emotional freedom to fully enjoy their lives. That is why Jeff created TotalSelf Counseling and Fitness. His approach to health includes psychotherapy, personal training, and nutrition counseling.

> ### Jeff Fine's Current Passion
>
> To expand my private practice providing psychotherapy, personal training, and nutrition counseling into a group practice with multiple practitioners in each discipline.

Jeff has a bachelor's degree in psychology from Syracuse University and two master's degrees (in clinical social work and nutrition) from New York University. He also completed an advanced training program in hypnosis at the New York Milton H. Erickson Society for Psychotherapy and Hypnosis. He then earned an advanced certificate in exercise science and personal training from the Swedish Institute, and he is a certified personal trainer from the National Strength and Conditioning Association. Jeff is a Crossfit trainer, has Crossfit certifications in barbell and Olympic lifting, and is a certified sports performance coach through USA Weightlifting. His published papers include "An Integrated Approach to Nutrition Counseling" (*Topics in Clinical Nutrition*) and "The Myth of Dieting" (*Hudson River Journal*).

Prior to opening TotalSelf Counseling and Fitness, Jeff maintained a full-time private practice in New York City. Past professional experience includes serving as a senior consultant to the New York City Department of Mental Health, teaching as an adjunct instructor at New York University's Department of Nutrition and Food Studies, and working in progressive, culturally diverse inpatient and outpatient settings.

Jeff resides in Westchester County, New York, with his wife Kerry.

Career Reflections

"My passion has always been to help as many people as possible optimize their physical and emotional health. I feel fortunate that over the past 20 years I have had the opportunity to do just that. I believe that the therapeutic relationship with a client is the most important agent of change. I also believe in the healing powers of laughter, humor, and exercise. With sensitivity and compassion, I try to use the full extent of my comprehensive education, training, and professional experience in the disciplines of psychotherapy, personal training, and nutrition counseling to help individuals, couples, families, and groups struggling with emotional, relational, behavioral, or physical problems.

"I learned early on that the path to a fulfilling and rewarding career includes the right mix of dogged determination, focus, planning, an open mind, and the ability to think out of the box. Through proactive networking I was able to create a wide range of new and exciting professional opportunities.

Jeff Fine's Words of Wisdom

- First, ask yourself what you need to feel fulfilled professionally.
- Second, ask yourself what the clients you choose to work with need you to know to help them. Repeat every three to six months for the rest of your career.

"As an adjunct instructor at New York University's Department of Nutrition, Food Studies, and Public Health, I began teaching a course I created, Nutrition Counseling Theory and Practice. As an outgrowth of teaching, I networked with NYU's Work, Life, and Wellness Services and began giving stress management workshops, and also developed and ran a focused support group called The Three Pillars—Mind, Body, and Food: A Non-Diet Approach to Permanent Weight Loss.

"For the practicing nutrition professional, I began offering workshops approved by the American Dietetic Association for continuing education credits, such as 'Beyond Diagnosis: The Person Behind the Eating Disorder,' and 'How to Start and Build Your Private Practice.' I also supervised NYU nutrition students interning at the Juilliard School for Music and Dance and gave workshops (stress management, eating disorders) to the Julliard student body. Needless to say, these opportunities also generated many patient referrals for my private practice."

Internet Communications: Kathleen M. Zelman, MPH, RD

Biography

Kathleen M. Zelman, MPH, RD, is a nutrition and communications consultant in private practice in Atlanta specializing in food, health, and nutrition communications for consumer and health professional audiences. She is also the director of nutrition for WebMD Health, where she serves as the professional expert for the company and online weight-loss program, and writes educational and motivational content on topics related to diet, health, and nutrition. Kathleen has over 20 years of media experience, including cohosting a weekly radio program and serving for 12 years as a national spokesperson for the

American Dietetic Association. She received her master's degree in public health from Tulane University and her bachelor of science from Montclair State University. Previous steps in her career included working as a clinical dietitian and in private practice, being an instructor at Georgia State University and assistant professor of nutrition at St. Mary's Dominican College, and serving as dietetic internship director at Ochsner Medical Institutions. She has also partnered with chefs Emeril Lagasse and Paul Prudhomme, and her media experience has included appearances on CNN, *Good Morning America*, NBC Nightly News, CBS Evening News, and *ABC World News*, and in the *Wall Street Journal* and the *New York Times*.

> **Kathleen Zelman's Current Passion:**
>
> Network with professionals around the globe.

GIVING BACK TO THE PROFESSION

In addition to her work as ADA media spokesperson, Kathleen's contributions to the dietetics profession have included:

- Louisiana Dietetic Association state media representative
- Director-at-large, ADA Board of Directors
- Georgia delegate, ADA House of Delegates
- Past trustee, Georgia Dietetic Foundation

Career Reflections

"All my life I wanted to be a ballerina, and when my father convinced me that the career of a dancer was short-lived, I started looking for a career that involved physical fitness. I took a basic nutrition course and was immediately inspired to learn all about food, nutrition, and its impact on fitness and health. Throughout my college career, I never looked back and always enjoyed the learning process so much so that later, I would even return to the classroom as an educator.

"As an educator, I loved watching the students grow in their knowledge, maturity, and commitment to dietetics. My passion for learning and students kept me in education for eight more years until I branched out into private practice.

"I also served as the Louisiana Dietetic Association state media representative for several years, then became an ADA media spokesperson and served in that role for 12 years. The exposure and experience as a media spokesperson opened doors to exciting travel and work opportunities. It allowed me to focus my career and develop new skills as a speaker, moderator, writer, and media trainer.

> ### Kathleen Zelman's Words of Wisdom
>
> - If you love what you do, you will be rewarded with a fabulous career and the great satisfaction that comes from helping others.
> - Keep challenging yourself to grow and learn, and seek opportunities for professional advancement.

"My latest career development came as a result of a phone call from WebMD, which I naturally thought was for an interview but turned out to be for a work opportunity. My role is as a professional expert for the company. I write features, expert reviews, review nutrition-related content for accuracy, develop educational material used on the site, serve as senior nutrition correspondent covering meetings and filing news reports, and perform any other tasks that have a nutritional component. I love working with folks who are savvy in information technology and who have taught me an enormous amount about computers and technology.

"Throughout my career, I have firmly believed in giving back to my profession. On a local, state, and national level, I have held numerous offices and positions. It is with great pleasure that I volunteer to serve the profession, and I must admit, the networking and friendships that have grown from my volunteer work is the greatest reward."

Latino Nutrition:
Malena Perdomo, MS, RD, CDE

Biography

Malena Perdomo, MS, RD, CDE, is an affiliate professor of nutrition in the Department of Health Professions at Metropolitan State College of Denver, Colorado, and has community, clinical, and research experience. She undertook a government nutrition internship in Panama, which enabled her to become the 126th nutritionist in her country in 1995. Her background also includes work for Kaiser Permanente Colorado, the WIC program in Nashville and Denver, community programs such as Children with Special Needs, translating nutrition materials into Spanish for various organizations; and diabetes research for Latina women with type 2 diabetes.

> **Malena Perdomo's Current Passion**
>
> Continue to help Latino communities through nutrition education, utilize media channels to promote healthful eating, and become a leader in diversity within ADA.

Malena is also a television media talent who appears on a Spanish- and English-language TV health show that airs in Colorado, where she takes part in recipe development, gives nutrition advice on healthy eating and exercise to Latinos, and is currently developing a cookbook related to the TV show. She is honored to serve as the Latino Nutrition Spokesperson for the American Dietetic Association. Malena lives in Denver with her two children, Alexander and Max.

Career Reflections

"I always knew I wanted to make food a big part of my life. I believe my inspiration came from my father, an entomologist, who introduced me to the field of agriculture. Applying for internships in the U.S. while I was in Panama was a challenge. But it was worth it.

"The dietetics profession has given me the chance to work in various positions and utilize my creativity and technical and media skills. I have learned about creating and writing recipes, using software to create nutrition information and patient educational materials, and creating nutritional messages for radio and television shows that are fun, easy to do, and inspirational.

"I have made myself known as the Latin foods expert, but I am always learning something new. My patients come from all backgrounds and different countries such as Colombia, Mexico, and Peru, as well as Puerto Rico. It is such a broad topic, and there is so much for us to learn from one another. I tell my students that every time I teach in my community I learn something new. I feel that I take more from them than they take from me.

"In my kitchen, I try new Latino recipes to experiment with local flavors and foods.

"Nutrition is like a box of many specialties, and there are so many to choose from. My box is full of community engagement, teaching students, and working with the media, and they are all connected in my practice. I can't decide to do one thing in nutrition yet, because I love everything that I am doing. Helping people is what really motivates and drives my passion to teach others."

Malena Perdomo's Words of Wisdom

- Cultural competence in nutrition should involve learning about foods and knowing how to prepare them, especially traditional dishes.
- When teaching in the community, I use a lot of visuals—such as food models, real foods, and food labels—and interactive group discussion, conversations, and experiential activities (eating is one of them).

Media and Nutrition:
Carolyn O'Neil, MS, RD

Biography

As a noted nutrition expert and television personality, Carolyn O'Neil, MS, RD, spreads her refreshing food philosophy, "The more you know, the more you can eat!" She is president of O'Neil Nutrition Communications in Atlanta, Georgia, and an award-winning author and journalist who reported on food and health at CNN for nearly 20 years. Other highlights of her career have included being the AOL Diet and Fitness Coach, writing a column for the *Atlanta Journal-Constitution,* and appearing as "The Lady of the Refrigerator," a recurring nutrition expert on Alton Brown's Food Network program, *Good Eats.* She coauthored *The Dish on Eating Healthy and Being Fabulous!* (Simon & Schuster, Atria Books), which won Best Health and Nutrition Book at the World Food Media awards. Carolyn has a master's degree in nutrition and communication from Boston University (1980) and an undergraduate degree in foods and nutrition from Florida State University (1976), and she served her dietetic internship at the Veteran's Administration Hospital in San Diego. Carolyn lives in Atlanta and has two children, Jack and Katie.

> ### Carolyn O'Neil's Current Passion
>
> Continue to raise the visibility of RDs as "the food and nutrition experts" in mass media print, broadcast, online, and social media outlets; and write another book.

Awards and Honors

Carolyn's CNN television reporting on food, nutrition, and cuisine earned three James Beard Foundation awards, and she was the first dietitian to be inducted into the James Beard *Who's Who in Food and Beverage*. The American Heart Association, ADA, and the National Restaurant Association have also presented O'Neil with awards for food and nutrition education.

Career Reflections

"Each time I tell someone I am a registered dietitian, I enjoy seeing their reaction. Through the years the response and the facial expressions have changed. In the 1980s, when I first started practicing, people would ask, 'What's that? Is that like a nutritionist?' And I'd have to go through some long explanation of how RDs go through more formal academic and clinical training than most people who just say they're a nutritionist. Then they'd say, 'Oh, so you work in a hospital.' I'd go on with my story and say, 'Well, no I don't. I like working in preventive health. You know, to get people the diet and nutrition information they need so they don't end up in the hospital.' That's when they'd laugh a bit and respond, 'Oh, don't look when I eat this brownie.' Being a dietitian at a dinner party was like being a minister in a bar!

> ### Carolyn O'Neil's Words of Wisdom
>
> - "Make is simple. Make it memorable. Make it inviting to look at. Make it fun to read." —Leo Burnett, advertising icon
> - If you enjoy what you're doing, it's not work. It's play.

"Jump forward to now. It's amazing when I tell people today that I'm a registered dietitian and the majority of people respond, 'Oh, that's really great.' And they launch into questions about their personal diet needs. 'What about this gluten-free thing?' 'What do you think about low-carb diets?' 'Do you buy acai berry juice?' Dietitians have emerged with a new image as nutrition experts who are food savvy and ready to share valuable and trustworthy personalized diet advice. OK, a lot of folks still try to hide their brownies."

Media and Fitness:
Felicia D. Stoler, DCN, MS, RD, FACSM

Biography

A registered dietitian and exercise physiologist, Felicia D. Stoler, DCN, MS, RD, FACSM, comes to the health and wellness field after a career at ABC News in New York City, before which she worked as a paralegal. Today, Felicia is a sought-after nutrition and fitness expert for conferences, TV, radio, newspapers, and magazines. In her career she has been an adjunct professor at Brookdale Community College, host of the second season of TLC's *Honey We're Killing the Kids!,* and nutrition coordinator for the ING New York City Marathon. Her media experience has included work with Ovaltine, *Dateline NBC's* first Weight Loss Challenge, Nike, GNC, Unilever, Cargill, Florida Department of Citrus, Nesquik, Eli Lilly, Milk Pep, National Dairy Council, Sirius Satellite Radio, and more.

> **Felicia Stoler's Current Passion**
>
> Being open-minded about adapting my options to the opportunities that present themselves to me based upon needs and demands.

Felicia holds a double master's degree in nutrition and exercise physiology from Teachers College, Columbia University, and completed her doctorate in clinical nutrition at the University of Medicine and Dentistry of New Jersey, where her research in work site wellness demonstrated that changes in nutrition and physical activity can improve measured health outcomes.

Giving Back to the Profession

Felicia currently serves in leadership roles for the American Dietetic Association, American College of Sports Medicine (ACSM), and the New Jersey Council on Physical Fitness and Exercise. Her appointments have included:

- Delegate, ADA House of Delegates
- President, media representative, and publicity chair, New Jersey Dietetic Association
- Vice president, treasurer, and secretary, Greater New York chapter of ACSM
- Fellow, ACSM

Career Reflections

"I laugh when people tell me it is too late to change careers. I had two totally different careers before I turned 30 and will have spent the entire decade of my 30s in graduate school. How did I come to be in this field? One day, I spoke with someone at ABC News who told me that a master's degree in journalism was a dime a dozen. She suggested that I become an authority in a field that I was passionate about and see if I could find a way to bring it back to media.

"I decided to apply to the program at Teachers College, Columbia University, because I was interested in nutrition and exercise as integral parts of the health and wellness equation. I was very intimidated by the amount of hard science required for nu-

Felicia Stoler's Words of Wisdom

- Nutrition and exercise are the least expensive, least invasive, and most effective ways to prevent and treat diseases.
- Give back to the community; a candle loses nothing by lighting other candles.

trition and exercise physiology, so I spent the next four years working my fingers to the bone.

"I often say to others, consider how you measure success—is it money, personal satisfaction, how your peers perceive you, or your impact on society? For me, they are all important. I have worked very hard to get everything that I have achieved. It is definitely tough balancing a career and family. While I am confident in my knowledge base, I want to emphasize that we must stay current with the research in our field and in other health-related disciplines.

"I am very lucky that I love what I do! Every day is different and above all, I am passionate about my work—and it shows. A palm reader once said, 'What you do now for work, you would do even if you weren't paid to do it.'"

Nutrition Support: M. Patricia (Trisha) Fuhrman MS, RD, FADA, CNSD

Biography

Trisha Fuhrman, MS, RD, FADA, CNSD, is a nutrition support and renal dietitian, and National Director of Nutrition for DCRX Infusion, in Sunrise, Florida. Highlights of her resume include liver transplant dietitian at Ochsner Medical Foundation, chair of dietetics at Jewish Hospital College of Nursing and Allied Health in St. Louis, clinical director of nutrition support at Saint Louis University Hospital, dietitian at Coram Healthcare, and coeditor of *RenaLink*. She has published journal

> **Trisha Fuhrman's Current Passion**
>
> Hone my skills in nutrition support and renal nutrition, sharpen my business acumen, and continue my professional involvement in ADA, ASPEN, and NKF/CRN.

articles and book chapters and lectured extensively on the topic of nutrition support.

Trisha's undergraduate degree is from Nicholls State University in Thibodaux, Louisiana. Her dietetic internship was done at Alton Ochsner Medical Foundation in New Orleans, and her master of science in nutrition and dietetics is from Saint Louis University.

Honors and Awards

Trisha has received numerous awards for excellence, including the 2002 American Dietetic Association Award for Excellence in Clinical Nutrition Practice, 2002 Dietitians in Nutrition Support Distinguished Service Award, and the Missouri Governor's Award for Excellence in Teaching.

Giving Back to the Profession

As a leader in her field, Trisha has served in numerous leadership roles for ASPEN, the American Dietetic Association, the National Kidney Foundation (NKF), and the Council on Renal Nutrition (CRN) of NKF. Among her accomplishments are the following:

- Member, National Kidney Foundation Council on Renal Nutrition
- ASPEN Board of Directors
- Chair, ASPEN Governance Task Force, Environmental Scan Task Force
- Nominating Committee, ASPEN
- Chair, ASPEN 2010 Interdisciplinary Review Course
- ADA Director-at-large
- ADA Professional issues delegate
- ADA Position Paper Committee
- Director for the ADA House Leadership Team
- ADA Board of Directors

- Speaker for the ADA House of Delegates
- Cochair of the St Louis Council on Renal Nutrition
- Member of the CME/CE Editorial Review Board for the National Kidney Foundation

Career Reflections

"I have attempted throughout my career to be visible, vocal, and vital as a member of the dietetics profession and as a member of the medical team. My success comes from not only my own efforts but from the support of my colleagues, friends, and family. As registered dietitians, we need to seize the career, political, research, and philanthropic opportunities available to advance the profession.

"Through my committee involvement in ASPEN, I met Virginia Herrmann, MD, who became a valuable mentor. It is a tremendous career boost to have a physician as an advocate—supporting and promoting the dietitian's expertise and professional goals.

"As important as paid employment is for professional growth and development, involvement in professional organizations is vital for my personal success and fulfillment. My involvement in ASPEN, ADA, NKF, and CRN provided many opportunities to hone leadership skills, and present and publish. Throughout my professional volunteerism I have enjoyed mentoring, professional growth, collegiality, and enduring friendships. Do not underestimate the personal benefits and rewards that come from professional involvement.

> ### Trisha Fuhrman's Words of Wisdom
>
> - Be alert to the professional opportunities around you and respond with your time and talents, when possible.
> - I spend my personal time on manuscripts, presentations, and other volunteer activities for professional organizations, and I have no regrets and would not dream of changing where I am or how I got here!

"I have been fortunate to have been honored by my peers. However, you cannot sit back and wait for others to recognize your talents and skills. Blow your own horn! Make sure your boss and colleagues know when you accomplish a personal or professional goal. Always maintain an updated resume/CV, since you never know when that professional accomplishment will lead to more presentations, research, publication, career opportunities, and organizational involvement."

Oncology Nutrition: Veronica McLymont, MS, RD, CDN

Biography

Known for her early advocacy of the American Dietetic Association's Nutrition Care Process and Model (NCP), which emphasizes nutrition diagnosis and a standardized process for nutrition documentation, Veronica McLymont, MS, RD, CDN, is the director of food and nutrition services at Memorial Sloan-Kettering Cancer Center, New York, New York, where she developed evidence-based clinical nutrition practice guidelines and integrated nutrition screening into adult and pediatric initial assessment tools. Her past experience included time as assistant director of dietetics at St. Barnabas Hospital in the Bronx, New York; chief clinical dietitian at Memorial Sloan-Kettering; and manager of clinical nutrition and patient services at Memorial Sloan-Kettering.

> **Veronica McLymont's Current Passion**
>
> I hope to be able to provide more consultative services to other entities and publish more outcomes and consumer-related materials.

Veronica strongly believes in patient-centered care and that it optimizes patient outcomes. She holds a master's degree in nutrition from Hunter College and is a doctoral candidate at the University of Maryland Eastern Shore.

Giving Back to the Profession

Among Veronica's contributions to the food and nutrition profession are the following:

- Nominating Committee member, New York State Dietetic Association
- President of the Westchester/Rockland Dietetic Association
- Chair, Nominating Committee for the Clinical Nutrition Management DPG
- Author, nutrition chapter for the textbook *Cancer Rehabilitation: Principles and Practice* (Stubbfield & O'Dell, 2009)

Career Reflections

"It has been a long and exciting journey. During my final semester in high school, my teacher invited the only dietitian in my hometown to speak to us about careers. She was a beacon of light for me. Coming from a small town, I'd never heard about what dietitians do, and she made me curious enough to pursue a career in dietetics.

"In my first job as a clinical dietitian, I worked diligently and exceeded my quota for assessments. My boss noticed and reassigned me to the outpatient clinic, where I worked independently. Networking with the physicians and nurses in the clinic established me as the nutrition expert. Just about every position I've held since then has been due in part to a professional connection.

"Meeting the unique nutrition requirements of the oncology patient can be challenging. Cancer and its therapies can alter nutritional status and compromise patient outcomes. One of my biggest accomplishments was collaborating with our dynamic team in developing and launching a groundbreaking room service meal-delivery program to address these concerns.

"I have utilized my years of experience to help improve patient service standards and continually work to improve patient satisfaction. I use the wealth of knowledge gained over my years of experience at Memorial Sloan-Kettering to translate best practices into standard practice.

"I believe that as leaders, dietetics professionals can go very far. Along the way they must help those who follow to aspire and achieve heights that help meet their own personal mission as well as those of the profession and their organizations."

Veronica McLymont's Words of Wisdom

- Pursue your passion.
- Be a role model . . . you're always on stage.

Publishing: Regina Ragone, MS, RD

Biography

Regina Ragone, MS, RD, food director for *Family Circle*, brings more than 20 years of nutrition expertise to the magazine. She has also been assistant manager at the Global Consumer Food Center of the Campbell Soup Company. Her previous publishing positions included an internship at *Restaurant Business Magazine*, employment at a small restaurant trade magazine, food editor for *Prevention* magazine; columnist ("In the Kitchen with Regina") and nutritionist for *Family Circle*, food editor at *Weight Watchers* magazine and the Weight Watchers Publishing Group, and test kitchen director for *Ladies' Home Journal*. She also worked as a public school foodservice dietitian, and she was a vice president at both Hunter Public Relations and

Regina Ragone's Five-Year Goal

To expand my role as food director of *Family Circle* into other multimedia brand extensions.

Ogilvy Public Relations. She is author of *Win the Fat War* cookbook and *Decadent Diabetic Desserts*, and coauthor of *Meals That Heal.*

Regina received her master's degree in nutrition from Queens College and her bachelor's in nutrition and foods from New York University. She resides in New York City, where she can enjoy a wide range of culinary experiences.

GIVING BACK TO THE PROFESSION

Regina is a member of the American Dietetic Association, the International Association of Culinary Professionals, the Association of Food Journalists, the New York Women's Culinary Alliance, and Les Dames d'Escoffier.

Career Reflections

"My nutrition training began in second grade when the school nurse sent me home with a note saying I had to lose weight. My mom stepped in, and without making me feel bad taught me what I needed to know to get into shape. I was hooked!

"Fast forward 10 years, and I enrolled in my mom's alma mater, New York University. I loved all of the nutrition classes I took, and I also loved food. I was torn between being a dietitian or a chef. I wanted to teach others about nutrition, but I also wanted people to know they could eat great food and still be healthy. I started reading *Gourmet, Bon Appetit,* and *Food & Wine* magazines. This was what I wanted to do—write about food, but healthy food. There was no place for someone with

> ### Regina Ragone's Words of Wisdom
>
> - Have a vision of where you want to go and write it down; I look back at the things I wrote down, and I have achieved them!
> - No one expects you to know everything, and others have more respect for you when you ask for their expertise.

my type of background, so when a friend I'd kept in touch with from NYU was offered an associate food editor position for a start-up magazine, she went for it and offered me the chance to work with her, if I was willing to take the risk. It was scary, but I jumped, and my life was never the same.

"Since then I have worked with several consumer publications as well as a nutritionist for two public relations companies. Every time I made a change it was difficult, and there was always a learning curve. I've had to tap into many of the nutrition contacts I've made through the years to help me. I am grateful for all of the support from my colleagues in every step of my journey and am excited to see where we're all headed."

Private Practice Nutrition: Cynthia Sass, MPH, MA, RD, CSSD

Biography

Owner of Sass Consulting Services, Inc., Cynthia Sass, MPH, MA, RD, CSSD, is a *New York Times* best-selling author and nationally known registered dietitian and health educator. She has been quoted as a nutrition and health expert in dozens of national publications and has appeared as a guest on several national radio and television shows, including *Today, Good Morning America, The Early Show, Rachael Ray, The Biggest Loser,* and others. She has served as a consultant for a cooking show, vegan workshops, professional sports teams (including the Philadelphia Phillies and Tampa Bay Rays), and for a grocery chain (recording podcasts and providing store tours). As a freelancer, she has written for *Ladies' Home Journal, Woman's Day,*

> **Cynthia Sass's Current Passion**
>
> To continue doing the things I enjoy most and seek new opportunities and adventures in the nutrition communications arena.

Family Circle, Prevention, Fitness, Shape, Self, More, Women's Health, Cooking Light, Eating Well, and many other publications. Cynthia has also been nutrition director and Grocery Guru for *Prevention* magazine and contributing editor and weight-loss coach for *Shape* magazine.

Cynthia was a national media spokesperson for the American Dietetic Association for six years and one of the first dietitians to become board certified as a specialist in sports dietetics. She maintains a private practice in Manhattan, where she works with individuals, couples, and families.

Cynthia has a bachelor's degree in nutrition/dietetics (summa cum laude) and a master's degree in nutrition science with a concentration in community counseling, both from Syracuse University. She also earned a master's degree in public health with a concentration in community and family health education at the University of South Florida.

Career Reflections

"I'm one of the fortunate people who entered college knowing what I wanted to 'be.' I always had a passion for both health and food. I loved going to the farmers' market and grocery store with my mother, I devoured health information from women's magazines, and when I found 'dietitian/nutritionist' in a health occupations book, I was hooked. When I graduated with my first master's degree, I wrote my long-term professional goals in a journal. I wanted to be in private practice, write, and be involved with media and public speaking. Ten years later, I am succeeding in each of those areas. I believe that my accomplishments are rooted in my enthusiasm for this field and a healthy work ethic.

"Throughout my career, I've worked hard to tactfully educate physicians, therapists, fitness professionals, clients, and the media about my professional role and abilities. Doing so has resulted in a level of

Cynthia Sass's Words of Wisdom

- Nutrition is one of the most dynamic and diverse fields to work in because food and nutrition are linked to nearly every aspect of life at every age, so there are unlimited opportunities to pursue if you are creative and entrepreneurial.
- Never forget or doubt your knowledge and skills—a registered dietitian is the premier food and nutrition expert!

respect and understanding that generates referrals and media inquiries. Dietitians are scientifically trained, well-credentialed professionals with 'big picture' knowledge. In a fad-crazy, quick-fix world, I sometimes feel like I'm swimming against the current, but faith in my knowledge and training keeps me grounded.

"I was recently at a dietetics meeting and was introduced to a new colleague as a nontraditional dietitian. It made me smile but also made me think, 'Is the definition of nontraditional becoming traditional?' I know lots of dietitians who are involved in unique projects, far outside the walls of a hospital or long-term care facility.

"In this field, we can be as inventive as we want to be, and there is enough work to go around for all of us. I believe that if you have a passion for this field, you will love what you do and do it well. As a result, you'll enjoy being active in shaping the profession, and many opportunities will come your way."

Sports Nutrition: Julie H. Burns, MS, RD, CCN

Biography

Julie H. Burns, MS, RD, CCN, is founder of SportFuel, Inc., and Eat Like the Pros, an integrative sports nutrition consulting company and organic meal delivery service. Past and current clients include the

Chicago Blackhawks, Chicago White Sox, Chicago Bears, Chicago Bulls, Northwestern University's varsity teams, Next Level Performance, and individual pro and elite athletes.

Julie earned her bachelor's degree in nutrition and dietetics from the University of Illinois at Urbana-Champaign (1983), and master's in clinical nutrition from the Massachusetts General Hospital Institute of Health Professions (1987). She is a registered and licensed dietitian in Illinois and is a Board Certified Clinical Nutritionist (CCN and IACCN), with experience in clinical research (working with Dr. Michael Davidson), public speaking, and public relations consulting. She has written chapters for multiple books on sports nutrition.

> ### Julie Burns's Current Passion
>
> To continue designing and providing services and products through SportFuel, Inc., a sports nutrition company, and Eat Like the Pros, an organic meal delivery service.

GIVING BACK TO THE PROFESSION

Among Julie's contributions to dietetics are the following:

- Executive Committee, Sports, Cardiovascular, and Wellness Nutrition (SCAN) DPG
- Member, SCAN and Dietitians in Integrative and Functional Medicine DPGs
- Member, Chicago, West Suburban, and Illinois Dietetic Associations
- Member, the International Association of Clinical Nutritionists, the American College of Sports Medicine, and the Weston A. Price Foundation
- Gatorade Sport Science Institute's Sports Nutrition Advisory Board

Career Reflections

"I began my studies as a chemistry major and thought I wanted to be a physician, like my grandfather. I was a nurse's aid while in high school and enjoyed working in health care. During my sophomore year in college, my mother (who was also attending college!) took a nutrition course and loved it. She encouraged me to do the same. Mothers really often do know best—and I soon changed my major to nutrition and dietetics.

"Growing up, I enjoyed both playing and watching sports. During college, a friend of mine gave me *The Athlete's Kitchen,* written by Nancy Clark, a sport's dietitian in Boston. I was so excited to read and learn of the link between nutrition and sports performance that I decided to apply for my internship in Boston at Massachusetts General Hospital (MGH), where Nancy had completed her program. I was accepted to the combined internship/master's program at the MGH Institute of Health Professions and did some concentrated work in exercise physiology.

Julie Burns's Words of Wisdom

- If you are passionate about helping people achieve health and wellness through food, then this is the perfect career path for you.
- "Let food be thy medicine and medicine be thy food." —Hippocrates

"When I finished my master's degree, I returned home to Chicago and started working in clinical research with Dr. Michael Davidson, a young and gifted cardiologist who was starting a research center, where I honed counseling, marketing, and budgeting skills that have been instrumental in running my businesses today. Dr. Davidson knew I was passionate about sports nutrition and recommended me to the Chicago Blackhawks when they called asking for a referral.

"My approach to nutrition has changed quite a bit since I began my career in the late 1980s, in large part due to my daughters' multiple food allergies. I found that a holistic approach to eating and living was helpful in enhancing our entire family's heath. I now use laboratory testing, homeopathic remedies, and food-based supplements to devise comprehensive plans for performance wellness."

Supermarket Nutrition: Maggie Moon, MS, RD

Biography

Currently working as corporate nutritionist for the New York City–based online grocery retailer FreshDirect, Maggie Moon, MS, RD, helps customers find the healthful foods they're seeking online (www.freshdirect .com). In her corporate role, she initiates, drives, and manages projects that promote public health. As a nutrition writer, Maggie writes for a range of audiences through peer-reviewed journals, trade magazines, and consumer publications. Her writings have been published in *Today's Dietitian, IDEA Fitness Journal, Nutrition Today, Big Apple Parent,* and other periodicals. She previously served as editor-in-chief of *Grapevine Student Newsletter* for the Columbia University Teachers College program in nutrition; was nutrition educator at Harlem RBI Afterschool Nutrition Workshops; and nutrition communications consultant to the USA Rice Federation, Tea Council of the USA, Unilever, FirstJuice, Cranberry Institute, and KIND bars.

> **Maggie Moon's Current Passion**
>
> Promote public health through supermarket initiatives, write a book, continue writing for magazines, mentor aspiring and new RDs, and serve in ADA leadership positions.

Maggie holds degrees from the University of California at Berkeley (bachelor's degree in English) and Columbia University Teachers College (master's degree in nutrition and education).

GIVING BACK TO THE PROFESSION

As an active ADA member, Maggie has served on the executive committee and Web site task force for the Sports, Cardiovascular, and Wellness Nutrition DPG. She has also been a dietetic intern preceptor as well as editor of the Greater New York Dietetic Association newsletter.

Career Reflections

"I always knew I loved food and words, but I never thought I'd love science. I came to nutrition by way of a degree in English literature, a brief career as a world-traveling professional Lindy Hopper, and a shoulder surgery–induced career change. It was in the latter stage that I recalled my fondness for food and health.

"I chose to apply to the Columbia University Teachers College program in nutrition because I saw an opportunity to work on upstream solutions such as nutrition education for high-need neighborhoods, be involved in public policy work, and design educational curricula that would teach kids about food from farm to fork. In short, I saw a confluence of my humanities background and my interest in nutrition. For me, the right thing to do was to apply to the one and only program I felt was a perfect fit; so I did, and am lucky they felt the same way.

"Beyond academics, what I value most are the connections I made with professors who became good friends and classmates who are now esteemed colleagues. A professor helped me get my very first job in New York City public schools. Later, a referral from a classmate

Maggie Moon's Words of Wisdom

- Be confident in your knowledge and skills while being humble and open to others' expertise.
- Showing people that eating healthy on a budget can also be delicious is a winning combination that really works!

helped me get my first job in nutrition communications, and mentors from that first job opened up opportunities for more freelance writing and volunteer opportunities with ADA.

"I feel grateful to be part of a profession that highly values mentorship. I'm still pretty new around here but am giving back in the small ways I can. I make myself open to calls and visits with prospective TC students and colleagues who want to know more about my work in supermarket nutrition, I take on dietetic interns, and I recently had the pleasure of referring a new RD for a position that she secured and is now enjoying."

Weight Loss:
Christopher R. Mohr, PhD, RD, CSSD

Biography

Christopher R. Mohr, PhD, RD, CSSD, is the owner and president of Mohr Results, Inc., a nutrition and fitness consulting company in Louisville, Kentucky. He is the sports nutritionist for Under Armour's Performance Training Council and is a media spokesperson for a number of companies. Christopher's expertise has been sought by celebrities, professional athletes, soccer moms, and everyone in between. He was consulting dietitian for the *New York Times* best-selling *LL Cool J's Platinum Workout* and has worked as a TV and radio nutrition and fitness expert, including for *Emeril Green*, with Chef Emeril Lagasse. He has also been a columnist for *Men's Fitness* magazine and published more than 500 articles for a variety of consumer publications, such as *Weight Watchers, Men's Health, Fitness, Prevention,* and more.

> **Christopher Mohr's Current Passion**
>
> Be the leading resource for honest and effective weight-loss information.

Christopher has bachelor's and master's degrees in nutrition from the Pennsylvania State University and the University of Massachusetts, respectively. He earned his PhD in exercise physiology from the University of Pittsburgh, and he is a registered dietitian and board certified specialist in sports dietetics.

Career Reflections

"I majored in nutrition at Penn State, but I didn't think I wanted to be a registered dietitian. To me, RDs only worked in hospitals, and I knew that was not of interest to me. When my classmates were getting ready to apply for dietetic internships, I remember telling my dad, 'I do not want to be a clinical dietitian and that's all RDs do.' He quickly came back with 'at least just apply. If you don't get in, then you won't have to worry about what you do with the credential. But when you have it, you can always use it to fall back on.'

"Like any 20 year old, I hated to admit my dad was right—but it was the most useful advice I'd heard. I applied to several internships, was matched at the University of Delaware, and now my expertise is sought out because I am a registered dietitian. It was one of the most important years of my career.

"While I was earning my PhD I was just one of two on our research team who was a dietitian, allowing me to be more involved from a nutrition front and therefore garner more experience. From a business perspective, it has clearly opened many doors for me, such as consulting with the Discovery Health Channel and Under Armour to

> **Christopher Mohr's Words of Wisdom**
>
> - You can create absolutely any future you want to create as a dietitian.
> - Stay current, understand the research, and never let anything get in the way of achieving everything that you want. Being a RD will help get you there.

being a sought-after expert in the fitness arena and working as a spokesperson for the trusted brands I work with.

"So while the initial conversations started with me suggesting there is nothing that could be done with the RD credential outside of working in a clinical setting, I now realize just how many opportunities have 'fallen' in my lap because I am a trusted nutrition expert."

A Closer Look

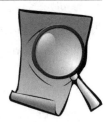

A Special Partnership: Tammy Lakatos Shames, RD, and Elysse ("Lyssie") Lakatos, RD —The Nutrition Twins

Biography

Tammy Lakatos Shames, RD, and Elysse ("Lyssie") Lakatos, RD, also known as "The Nutrition Twins," are registered dietitians and personal trainers who share more than identical features; they share a mission to help people improve their health through lifestyle-focused behavior modification. What began as a passion for bettering the way people feel inside and out morphed into the founding of an innovative nutrition company, The Nutrition Twins. This endeavor enables the twins to impact millions of people worldwide through a variety of media.

Tammy and Lyssie have become known for their unique approach to nutrition counseling, corporate lecturing, writing, media appearances, and consulting for multinational food companies. The Lakatos sisters have worked with over 200 corporations and serve as the exclusive nutritionists for NBC's celebrities and employees at Rockefeller Plaza in New York City.

Lyssie and Tammy drew from their experiences to coauthor *Fire Up Your Metabolism: 9 Proven Principles for Burning Fat and Losing Weight Forever* (Simon & Schuster). Their next book, *The Secret to Skinny: How Salt Makes You Fat, and the 4-Week Plan to Drop a Size and Get Healthier with Simple Low-Sodium Swaps* was released in the fall of 2009. In a venture with Day-Timer, they developed a Wellness Planner and Weight Management Planner, which they featured several times on QVC in early 2009.

The twins have been featured regularly as nutrition experts on the Discovery Health channel, Fox News Channel, NBC, Bravo, WABC-TV, WPIX-TV, CBS, The Learning Channel, FitTV, Oxygen Network, Life and Style, Court TV, *Fox & Friends*, and *Good Day New York*. Tammy and Lyssie were also featured in a special "makeover" show of *Queer Eye for the Straight Guy* in which they helped two "straight guys" to each lose 60 pounds.

Tammy and Lyssie have become sought-after contributors to many print and online publications. They have been featured on the cover of *Woman's World* magazine and have appeared in *Cosmopolitan, Self, Good Housekeeping, Vogue, InStyle, Woman's Day, Parents, First for Women, Oxygen, Muscle Media, OK!, Star Magazine, Fitness, Glamour, People, Health, O, Lifetime, Reader's Digest, The New York Daily News, Women's Health and Fitness, Remedy,* and *Family Circle* magazines. In addition, they have contributed to online resources including WebMD, MSN, WeightWatchers.com, Discovery Health (discovery.com), TLC.com, eDiets.com, and AOL Diet and Fitness. The twins have also been featured experts on numerous radio stations across the United States and around the world.

The twins have appeared as speakers for professional organizations, including the keynote speakers for the New Jersey Dietetic Association's annual meeting as well as featured presenters at the International Society of Sports Nutrition's annual conference.

Tammy and Lyssie reside in New York City, where they assist celebrities, professional athletes, and everyday people in attaining their personal health-related goals. For example, they helped the U.S. team prepare for Eco-Challenge, a grueling race that involves trekking, whitewater canoeing, horseback riding, sea kayaking, scuba diving, mountaineering, camelback riding, and mountain biking over a 300-mile course. Former soccer and speed skating competitors, the twins now enjoy running and pumping iron, and Tammy chases after her twin girls to keep fit. For more on the Nutrition Twins, go to their Web site (www.nutritiontwins.com).

Q & A with the Nutrition Twins

Kyle and Milton: Apart from your twin status, what makes you different from your competition?

Tammy: Good question. We actually have a lot of great competition, which we are thankful for since they motivate us and inspire us to work harder. I think the biggest thing that separates us is that we do not limit ourselves to just counseling or just seminars or just writing; we really love to do it all, so we do.

Lyssie: We really try to personalize everything that we do—whether it is a lecture that we give or an individual consult, it will have our own style in it. And although everyone's style is different, I think that our style of counseling/lecturing, etc., makes us different from our competition.

K & M: Did you both decide at the same time that you wanted to become dietitians?

Tammy: We always were very athletic and wanted to know what would make us perform better or run faster. We both thought that proper nutrition would probably be a key factor for us. Lyssie always tells me that she decided first to study nutrition and that I always just wanted to do what she did, but I beg to differ!

Lyssie: I always say I decided first, and since I am 17 minutes older, Tammy wanted to do whatever I did, so she followed and decided to immediately after me. However, we were both always intrigued by food and its link to health, and I think we both finalized our decision during our freshman year of college, when we were both getting a little taste of college life and trying to survive on dining hall food.

K & M: How has your nutrition education helped you as entrepreneurs?

Tammy: It has given me a solid foundation, which has given me the confidence to be an entrepreneur. Once you believe in yourself and are excited about helping others, the entrepreneur part is part of the package. Even though my nutrition education has helped me in that respect, I still learn something new about business all of the time.

Lyssie: I think the part of my education that contributed most to me as an entrepreneur was experiencing clinical, foodservice management, and community

rotations during my internship. I also spent six
weeks following a dietitian of my choice. I saw all of
the different avenues that one could take as a dietitian and I saw how each operated and how each
drove their business. I learned that there were several things that I enjoyed doing and that I wanted my
practice to incorporate each of those aspects.

K & M: Who helped you the most during your career?

Tammy: Actually, Lyssie has helped me more than anyone
else (although a lot of other mentors, including my
professors and my internship director, Debbie Clegg,
have helped me a lot, too).

Lyssie: Gosh, that's a tough one. There have been so many
people who have been so helpful in my career. But I
think that one of the most instrumental was Ansley
Hudson. I spent three weeks of my internship with
her. I had chosen to work with her. She was in private
practice in Charlotte, North Carolina. She was a consultant for the Carolina Panthers, numerous professional race car drivers, and other professional athletes. She worked in an office and as part of a team
with a sports agent and physical therapist/personal
trainer. It was a great setup. Ansley's practice included a lot of corporate wellness. She gave health fairs
and nutrition seminars to different corporations. She
allowed me to counsel professional athletes on my
own. This gave me the confidence to see I could do it
and that high-caliber athletes would listen to me and
respect me. She also let me lecture one of her corporate accounts. Furthermore, she was very open in
showing me how she ran her business and what it
takes to succeed. She was a very hard worker, and I
quickly realized that you have to be very motivated

and disciplined in order to succeed as an entrepreneur. I began my career by structuring it somewhat
like hers. And I also remember how much she helped
me, and I try to help other interns or people in the
profession as much as she did for me.

K & M: Tell us about your successful private practice.

Tammy: I view success as happiness and being excited about
waking up every morning and going to work. We love
what we do, every aspect of it. We counsel clients,
give corporate seminars, act as spokespeople, and
serve as experts for television, radio, and print outlets. No two days are ever the same. One day we may
see clients and give a seminar and the next day we
may film a TV show and work on a piece for a magazine. The variety keeps things really exciting for us.

Lyssie: Our practice is actually somewhat like Ansley's was,
since we modeled it after hers. We have clients who
see us individually. Originally, athletes were our primary clients and we networked with personal trainers and exchanged referrals with them. As time pro-
gressed, we started to have more weight-loss clients,
but also we started to see a lot of clients who wanted
basic disease prevention through nutrition (lower
cholesterol, etc.). We also provide corporate seminars ("lunch-and-learns" on any number of nutrition
topics) for many corporations in New York City. Also,
we offer 6-, 8-, and 10-week weight management,
heart-healthy, and general nutrition programs that
we developed for corporations. And lately, we have
also been doing a lot of media and TV appearances
in which we are featured as "nutrition experts." Every
day is different, which we really cherish.

K & M: How did you get hired as the exclusive nutritionists for NBC's celebrities and employees at Rockefeller Plaza?

Tammy: It was all about timing, having a good resume, and a lot of luck! We knocked on a lot of doors before this one opened.

Lyssie: We were persistently making cold calls trying to see if we could send our brochures to the right person at corporations who may possibly be interested in having us do our seminars for their employees. We thought we were calling GE (it had just merged with NBC), and it was the first call out of about 50 where someone actually picked up the phone, was friendly, and wanted us to come in and meet with them. From there, it was a matter of good timing—their past dietitian had just left and the last few people who tried to become the dietitians there really had ulterior motives (like dropping off their resumes for Conan O'Brien!). So, they were looking for dietitians who fit in well with the company and who truly had no ulterior motives. We had a four-hour interview that day and then got the position!

K & M: What motivates you?

Tammy: I am motivated by other hard-working dietitians and their success. I love watching other dietitians succeed—it excites me to know that others can achieve success, and I try to as well.

Lyssie: I am motivated by many things. I am motivated when I think there is someone who could really benefit from one of my services. For instance, if I meet someone who is struggling with their weight and needs and wants help, I become very motivated to help them in every way possible. I like the way it feels to help people, and this motivates me. Other dietitians also motivate me. I learn from other dietitians, and if I see that they are teaching their clients and using knowledge I do not have, I am very motivated to become more educated. Also, I think I am motivated by success. I want to be successful (for me, being successful is feeling as though I am continually growing and improving as a registered dietitian and as an entrepreneur). And I feel that if I am always trying to learn more and get more business opportunities, ultimately, that will create success for me, and that motivates me.

K & M: What was it like to work with the U.S. Eco-Challenge team in preparation for the 24-hour competition?

Tammy: Exciting! Athletes, especially those who are so focused on their goal, are so much fun to work with. They listen to every word that you say and follow every piece of advice; they want that extra edge. I love the respect they have for their nutritionist. Our advice is like gold to them, which is really great.

Lyssie: It was an amazing experience. It is an awesome feeling to have people who are so disciplined and are working toward a goal. It was also a fantastic learning experience for me as I truly witnessed that everyone responds differently to foods. I really saw that everyone must be approached as an individual rather than as a team when it comes to their nutrition. It was great to watch body composition change and performance improve as the athletes' diets improved.

K & M: How did you get your book contract with Simon & Schuster for *Fire Up Your Metabolism: 9 Proven Principles for Burning Fat and Losing Weight Forever?*

Tammy: We actually were fortunate enough to get a literary agent who was instrumental in helping us to get a great publisher. And although writing the book proposal (and of course writing the book) required a lot of work, it also involved a little bit of luck when it came to getting the book deal.

Lyssie: After we stumbled upon a literary agent who liked us and our idea, we had to make a proposal for our book. A literary agent submits your proposal to the different publishing houses, and having an agent helps to ensure that your work is actually considered/reviewed and that it just doesn't lie on a desk, never to be looked at. The houses that were interested in our book requested to meet with us and our agent. At that point, our agent told the houses that all offers must be in by a certain day and time so that we were not sitting around waiting. Simon & Schuster gave us the best offer for our book, and we really liked the editor we would be working with, so we chose them as our publisher.

K & M: You both have been featured regularly as the nutrition experts for many prominent media outlets. You both must have a media agent. What's the most important piece of advice you can give to anyone who wants to work with the media?

Tammy: It actually wasn't an agent who lined us up with these opportunities. It's all about networking and hard work. And persistence. And that's my advice to anyone who wants to work with the media . . . be persistent. Do not get discouraged. One day a door will open for you, and then many will follow. Do you know how many "no's" we got before we got a "yes"?

Lyssie: Do not give up. If you pitch an idea that you would like to write or talk about to a media outlet and you do not hear back from them, it doesn't necessarily mean that they aren't interested; it just means they are busy. And if they tell you outright that they are not interested in that idea, do not get discouraged— pitch a different one!

K & M: Looking back at it all, all your successes and experiences, what would you change?

Tammy: Hmm . . . good question. Not much. But I think I would have done an internship program that had a combined master's program.

Lyssie: The only things that I would change are financially related. When we moved from Atlanta to New York, we kept the same accountant, who really didn't know New York tax laws, and we wound up incurring major tax fees for paying them at the wrong quarterly times. I now know always to keep your accountant nearby! Also, I learned when it comes to your Web site, ask people who they use as a designer and then talk to other people who use that same designer to make sure he or she is easy to contact and makes changes and updates your site when necessary. We wasted a lot of money because it took three times to finally get a reliable and efficient designer.

K & M: Do you plan to attend graduate school? Why or why not?

Tammy: I would love to go to graduate school. I know it sounds cliché, but knowledge truly is power (not to mention, it gives you more credibility). Our field changes so much day to day with all of the new research, and it really is important to stay on top of it. I read everything that I can get my hands on, and it's still not enough. The only thing holding me back from graduate school is finding the time in a crazy work schedule (here I am, still working, and it is after 1 AM, and I have little twin daughters who will be up in a couple of hours).

Lyssie: Absolutely! I love learning and feel like I still want to learn so much more and feel like you can always learn more in this great, ever-changing field.

K & M: What do you both want to be doing in 10 years?

Tammy: To be honest, I love what I do now, and if I am still doing it in 10 years, I would be thrilled! I have a nice mix of private clients, corporate seminars, some spokesperson work, and TV gigs. If anything, I guess I would like to do more spokesperson work and more television. But I'm not complaining, life is good!

Lyssie: You know, this is a very strange question for me—I always know what I want and where I want to go. However, this career has been an amazing whirlwind (if you asked me five years ago what I would want to be doing in five years, I would have described what I am doing now) and as I am faced with so many different amazing opportunities, I would be thrilled if any pan out and each could take me into an entirely different future.

Afterword

Hi there, reader!

It's us, Kyle and Milton, again. If you're reading this, we hope it's because you've recently earned your RD credential and have kept this guide by your side along the way.

As we said at the start, we wish we'd had something like this book when we were learning the ropes. We hope we've made it easier for you to navigate your way to the RD credential and that you're now ready and energized to make the most of your career! Being a registered dietitian is a rewarding career choice, and we hope you love it as much as we do.

If you've taken our advice, you'll be volunteering for ADA any day now and putting your networking skills to good use, which means we'll run into each other soon enough. Though we are nearly 80,000 strong, the dietetics community is relatively small (in a good way). When you see us, please say hello!

We hope this guide has been a valuable companion to you. Good luck to you and thank you for all the good work you'll be doing in the name of nutrition!

Our best wishes,
—*Kyle and Milton*

Appendix A

Internet Resources

Chapter 1: Welcome to Dietetics!
- **American Dietetic Association (ADA)**: www.eatright.org
- **ADA Knowledge Center**: knowledge@eatright.org
- **Commission on Dietetic Registration (CDR)**: www.cdrnet.org

Chapter 2: Hitting the Books
- **Commission on Accreditation for Dietetics Education (CADE)**:
  www.eatright.org/CADE
- **CADE-accredited Coordinated Programs in Dietetics (CPDs)**:
  www.eatright.org/CADE-CP
- **CADE-accredited Didactic Programs in Dietetics (DPDs)**:
  www.eatright.org/CADE-DPD
- **CADE-accredited Dietetic Internships (DIs)**: www.eatright.org/CADE-DI

Chapter 3: The Nitty-Gritty Details of the Dietetic Internship

Application Information and Resources
- **ADA page of the D & D Digital Web site** (registration for computer matching
  with internships): https://www.dnddigital.com/ada/index.php
- **ADA Student Center**: www.eatright.org/students
- **CADE-accredited Dietetic Internships (DIs)**: www.eatright.org/CADE-DI
- **Dietetic Educators of Practitioners dietetic practice group** (source for
  standard dietetic internship application): www.depDPG.org

Financial Aid

- **Federal grants and loans information**: http://studentaid.ed.gov
- **Free Application for Federal Student Aid**: www.fafsa.ed.gov

Dietetics Student Blogs

AllAccessInternships.com has a list of dietetics student bloggers in the Links page of the Resources section.

Chapter 4: The Registration Examination for Dietitians

- **CDR Web site**: www.cdrnet.org
- **CDR e-mail**: CDR@eatright.org

Chapter 5: Secrets to Success: An Orientation for the New RD

CDR Resources

- **CDR's Professional Development Portfolio Guide**: www.cdrnet.org/pdrcenter
- **Credentials and certifications offered by CDR**: www.cdrnet.org/certifications

Top Nutrition Conferences

- **ADA Food and Nutrition Conference and Exhibition**: www.eatright.org/fnce
- **Clinical Nutrition Week**: www.nutritioncare.org
- **International Congress of Dietetics**: www.internationaldietetics.org/congress.aspx
- **National Restaurant Association**: http://show.restaurant.org
- **State Dietetic Association meetings**: www.eatright.org/affiliates (click Directory link for information about specific affiliate meetings)

ADA Resources

- **ADA Center for Professional Development** (includes continuing education listings): www.eatright.org/cpd
- **ADA Member Center**: www.eatright.org/members
- **ADA dietetic practice groups**: www.eatright.org/dpgs
- **ADA member interest groups**: http://www.eatright.org/migs
- **ADA state affiliate groups**: www.eatright.org/affiliates (also listed in Appendix C)

Other Nutrition-Related Groups and Resources

See also **Appendix B.**

- **American Association of Diabetes Educators**: www.aadenet.org
- **American College of Nutrition (ACN)**: www.americancollegeofnutrition.org
- **American Society for Nutrition**: www.nutrition.org
- **American Society for Parenteral and Enteral Nutrition (ASPEN)**: www.nutritioncare.org
- **Dietary Managers Association (DMA)**: www.dmaonline.org
- **School Nutrition Association (SNA)**: www.schoolnutrition.org
- **Society for Nutrition Education (SNE)**: www.sne.org
- **U.S. Food and Nutrition Information Center Professional and Career Resources section**: http://fnic.nal.usda.gov

Certifications from Beyond the ADA

- **American College of Sports Medicine (ACSM) certifications**: www.acsm.org
- **American Council on Exercise (ACE) certifications**: www.acefitness.org
- **Board Certified Advanced Diabetes Management**: www.nursingworld.org/ANCC
- **Certified Diabetes Educator**: www.ncbde.org
- **Certified Health Education Specialist**: www.nchec.org
- **Certified in Family and Consumer Sciences**: www.aafcs.org
- **Certified Nutrition Support Clinician**: www.nutritioncare.org
- **Certified Personal Trainer**: www.nasm.org
- **Certified Personal Trainer**: www.ncsf.org
- **Certified Professional in Healthcare Quality**: www.nahq.org
- **Certified Strength and Conditioning Specialist or NSCA-Certified Personal Trainer**: www.nsca-cc.org
- **International Board Certified Lactation Consultant**: www.iblce.org
- **National Certified Counselor**: www.nbcc.org

Resources for Writers

- **American Medical Writers Association**: www.amwa.org
- **FreelanceWriting.com**: www.freelancewriting.com

Chapter 6: Scoring Your First Gig and Beyond

Job Resources

- **Careerbuilder**: www.careerbuilder.com
- **Craigslist**: www.craigslist.org
- **Idealist**: www.idealist.org
- **IhireNutrition**: www.ihirenutrition.com
- **Indeed**: www.indeed.com
- **LinkedIn**: www.linkedin.com
- **Monster**: www.monster.com
- **Nutritionjobs**: www.nutritionjobs.com

Business Cards and Stationery

- **Overnightprints**: www.overnightprints.com
- **Vistaprint**: www.vistaprint.com

Salary Guides

- **Bureau of Labor Statistics**: www.bls.gov
- **Riley Guide**: www.rileyguide.com
- **Salary.com**: www.salary.com

Top Sources of Nutrition Information

- **American Institute for Cancer Research Newsletter**: www.aicr.org/publications
- *Berkeley's Wellness Letter*: www.berkeleywellness.com
- **Center for Human Nutrition Newsletter**: www.utsouthwestern.edu (search Center for Human Nutrition)
- *EdNet: National Food Safety Educator's Network*: www.foodsafety.gov/news /educators
- *Environmental Nutrition*: www.environmentalnutrition.com
- *Feeding Kids Newsletter*: www.nutritionforkids.com
- **Food and Nutrition Research Briefs**: www.ars.usda.gov/is/np/fnrb
- *Food Reflections Newsletter*: http://food.unl.edu/web/fnh/Food-reflections
- **Harvard Health Letters**: www.health.harvard.edu
- *Journal of the American Dietetic Association*: www.adajournal.org
- **Kansas State University Nutrition Extension** *Nutrition News*: www.ksre.ksu .edu/humannutrition (select Newsletters from Home page menu)
- **MCH (Maternal and Child Health) Research to Practice**: www.ncemch.org/research/diss.html#1

- **National Food Service Management Institute's *NFSMI Insight***: www.nfsmi.org
- **Nutrition Action Health Letter**: www.cspinet.org/nah
- **Nutrition and Your Child**: www.kidsnutrition.org
- ***Nutrition Insights***: www.cnpp.usda.gov/nutritioninsights.htm
- **The Johns Hopkins Medical Letter: Health After 50**: www.hopkinsafter50.com
- ***Today's Dietitian***: www.todaysdietitian.com
- **Tufts University Health & Nutrition Letter**: www.tuftshealthletter.com

Appendix B

Leading Nutrition- Related Organizations

American Dietetic Association
120 South Riverside Plaza, Suite 2000
Chicago, IL 60606-6995
Phone: 800/877-1600
www.eatright.org

American College of Nutrition
300 S. Duncan Avenue, Suite 225
Clearwater, FL 33755
Phone: 727/446-6086
E-mail: office@americancollegeof
nutrition.org
www.americancollegeofnutrition.org

American College of Sports Medicine
401 West Michigan Street
Indianapolis, IN 46202-3233
Mailing Address: PO Box 1440
Indianapolis, IN 46206-1440
Phone: 317/637-9200
www.acsm.org

American Diabetes Association
1701 North Beauregard Street
Alexandria, VA 22311
Phone: 800/342-2383
www.diabetes.org

American Heart Association
7272 Greenville Avenue
Dallas, TX 75231
Phone: 800/242-8721
www.heart.org

American Society for Parenteral and Enteral Nutrition (ASPEN)
8630 Fenton Street, Suite 412
Silver Spring, MD 20910
Phone: 301/587-6315
E-mail: aspen@nutr.org
www.nutritioncare.org

Dietitians of Canada
480 University Avenue, Suite 604
Toronto, ON, Canada M5G 1V2
Phone: 416/596-0857
www.dietitians.ca

Gerontological Society of America
1220 L Street NW, Suite 901
Washington, DC 20005
Phone: 202/842-1275
www.geron.org

Health Canada

Address Locator 0900C2

Ottawa, ON Canada K1A 0K9

Phone: 866/225-0709

E-mail: Info@hc-sc.gc.ca

www.hc-sc.gc.ca

Institute of Food Technologists

525 West Van Buren, Suite 1000

Chicago, IL 60607

Phone: 312/782-8424

E-mail: info@ift.org

www.ift.org

National Restaurant Association

1200 17th Street NW

Washington, DC 20036

Phone: 202/331-5900

or 800/424-5156

www.restaurant.org

Obesity Society

8757 Georgia Avenue, Suite 1230

Silver Spring, MD 20910

Phone: 301/563-6526

www.obesity.org

School Nutrition Association

120 Waterfront Street, Suite 300

National Harbor, MD 20745

Phone: 301/686-3100

E-mail:

servicecenter@schoolnutrition.org

www.schoolnutrition.org

Appendix C

State Dietetic Associations

Alabama Dietetic Association
Districts: Auburn, Birmingham, Eastern Shore, Mobile, Montgomery, North Alabama, Northeast, Northwest, Southeast, Tuscaloosa, Tuskegee
Web site: www.eatrightalabama.org

Alaska Dietetic Association
Districts: None
Web site: www.eatrightalaska.org

American Overseas Dietetic Association
Districts: None
E-mail: secretary@eatrightoverseas.org
Web site: www.eatrightoverseas.org

Arizona Dietetic Association
Districts: Central Arizona, Northern Arizona, Southern Arizona, Southwestern Arizona
E-mail: info@eatrightarizona.org
Web site: www.eatrightarizona.org

Arkansas Dietetic Association
Districts: Northwest Arkansas, Northeast Arkansas, Western Arkansas, Central Arkansas
E-mail: webmaster@arkansaseatright.org
Web site: www.arkansaseatright.org

California Dietetic Association
Districts: Bay Area, Northern Area, Coastal Tri-Counties, Los Angeles, San Diego, Central Valley, San Jose, Orange, Diablo Valley, Inland Empire
Web site: www.dietitian.org

Colorado Dietetic Association
Districts: Denver, Northern, Southern
E-mail: eatrightcolorado@gmail.com
Web site: www.eatrightcolorado.org

Connecticut Dietetic Association
Districts: None
E-mail: CDA_Secretary@dietetics.com
Web site: www.dietetics.com/cda

Delaware Dietetic Association
Districts: None
Web site: www.dedietassn.org

District of Columbia Metropolitan Area Dietetic Association
Districts: None
Web site: www.dcmada.org

Florida Dietetic Association
Districts: Broward, Orlando, Gainesville, Jacksonville, Miami, Tampa, Tallahassee, Pinellas, Palm Beach, West Florida, Panhandle, Cypress, Manasota, Southwest Florida, Space Coast
E-mail: info@eatrightflorida.org
Web site: www.eatrightflorida.org

Georgia Dietetic Association
Districts: Augusta, Coastal Empire, Columbus, Greater Atlanta, Middle Georgia, Northeast Georgia, Northwest Georgia, Southwest Georgia
E-mail: info@eatrightgeorgia.org
Web site: www.eatrightgeorgia.org

Hawaii Dietetic Association
Districts: None
Web site: www.eatrighthawaii.org

Idaho Dietetic Association
Districts: None
Web site: http://eatrightidaho.org

Illinois Dietetic Association
Districts: Capital, Central Illinois, Chicago, Eastern Illinois, Mississippi Valley, North Suburban, Rock River Valley, South Suburban, Southern Illinois, West Suburban
E-mail: headquarters@eatrightillinois.org
Web site: www.eatrightillinois.org

Indiana Dietetic Association
Districts: Central Indiana, East Central Indiana, Northeast Indiana, Northern Indiana, Northwest Indiana, Southeast Indiana, Southwest Indiana, West Central Indiana, Western Indiana
Web site: www.dietetics.com/ida

Iowa Dietetic Association
Districts: Hawkeye Area, Central Iowa, Mid-East Iowa, Midwest Iowa, Mississippi Valley, Northeast Iowa, Southwest Iowa, Upper Iowa
Web site: www.eatrightiowa.org

Kansas Dietetic Association
Districts: Kansas City, Kaw Valley, Tri Rivers, Western Kansas, Wichita, Southeast
E-mail: kda_exec@dietetics.com
Web site: www.dietetics.com/kda

Kentucky Dietetic Association
Districts: Bluegrass, Louisville, Northern Kentucky, Western Kentucky, Eastern Kentucky
Web site: www.kyeatright.org

Louisiana Dietetic Association
Districts: Shreveport, Northeast Louisiana, Central Louisiana, Southwest Louisiana, Arcadiana, Baton Rouge, Bayou, Southeast Louisiana, New Orleans
Web site: www.eatrightlouisiana.org

Maine Dietetic Association
Districts: None
Web site: www.eatrightmaine.org

Maryland Dietetic Association
Districts: None
Web site: www.eatwellmd.org

Massachusetts Dietetic Association
Districts: Cape Cod and the Islands,
Central Massachusetts, Northeast
Massachusetts, Southeast Massachusetts,
Western Massachusetts
Web site: www.eatrightma.org

Michigan Dietetic Association
Districts: Ann Arbor, Flint, Lansing,
Northern Michigan, Southeastern
Michigan, Southwest Michigan,
Tri-City, Upper Peninsula, Dietitians of
West Michigan
E-mail: mda.execdir@sbcglobal.net
Web site: www.eatrightmich.org

Minnesota Dietetic Association
Districts: Twin Cities, Head of the Lakes,
Northwest Minnesota, Rochester, South
Central Minnesota
Web site: www.eatrightmn.org

Mississippi Dietetic Association
Districts: Central, South Central, Gulf
Coast, Northeast, Northwest
Web site: www.eatrightmississippi.org

Missouri Dietetic Association
Districts: Kansas City, Southwest,
Southeast, Northwest, Northeast,
Central, South Central, St. Louis.
Web site: www.eatrightmissouri.org

Montana Dietetic Association
Districts: None
Web site:
www.montanadieteticassociation.org

Nebraska Dietetic Association
Districts: Central Nebraska, Lincoln,
North East, Omaha, West Central
Web site: www.eatrightnebraska.org

Nevada Dietetic Association
Districts: Northern Nevada, Southern
Nevada
Web site: www.nevadard.com

New Hampshire Dietetic Association
Districts: None
Web site: www.eatrightnh.org

New Jersey Dietetic Association
Districts: None
E-mail: njda@hq4u.com
Web site: www.eatrightnj.org

New Mexico Dietetic Association
Districts: Albuquerque, Southern New
Mexico
Web site: www.eatrightnm.org

New York State Dietetic Association
Districts: Greater New York, Long Island,
Westchester Rockland, Mid-Hudson,
Hudson Valley, Southern Tier, Mohawk
Regional, Central New York, Genesee,
Western New York
Web site: www.eatrightny.org

North Carolina Dietetic Association
Districts: Charlotte, Coastal, Durham-
Chapel Hill, Foothills, Greensboro, Ra-
leigh, Eastern, Twin City, Western
Web site: www.eatrightnc.org

North Dakota Dietetic Association
Districts: Bismarck-Mandan, Fargo-
Moorhead, Greater Grand Forks, James-
town-Valley City, Minot
Web site: www.eatrightnd.org

Ohio Dietetic Association
Districts: Greater Akron, Greater Cin-
cinnati, Cleveland, Columbus, Dayton,
Mahoning Valley, Mohican Area,
Northwest, Stark
E-mail: Info@EatRightOhio.org
Web site: www.eatrightohio.org

Oklahoma Dietetic Association
Districts: Southeast, Tulsa, Oklahoma
City, North Central, Southwest
E-mail: oknutrition@oknutrition.org
Web site: www.oknutrition.org

Oregon Dietetic Association
Districts: Willamette, Portland
E-mail: oda@quidnunc.net
Web site: www.eatrightoregon.org

Pennsylvania Dietetic Association
Districts: Central Pennsylvania, Lehigh
Valley, Northeast Pennsylvania, North-
west Pennsylvania, Philadelphia,
Pittsburgh
Web site: www.eatrightpa.org

Puerto Rico Chapter of ADA
Districts: None
Web site: www.adapr.2om.com

Rhode Island Dietetic Association
Districts: None
Web site: www.eatrightri.org

South Carolina Dietetic Association
Districts: Charleston, Catawba, Colum-
bia, Pee Dee, Piedmont
E-mail: eatrightsc@capconsc.com
Web site: www.eatrightsc.org

South Dakota Dietetic Association
District: Black Hills
Web site: www.eatrightsd.org

Tennessee Dietetic Association
Districts: Chattanooga, Knoxville, Mem-
phis, Nashville, Tri-Cities, Upper Cum-
berland, West Tennessee
Web site: www.eatright-tn.org

Texas Dietetic Association
Districts: Austin, Central Texas,
Dallas, El Paso, Houston, Mid East,
Panhandle, San Antonio, Texarkana, Big
Country, Corpus Christi, East Texas,
Fort Worth, Lubbock, North Texas, Rio
Grande, Tall Pines, West
E-mail: TDA@eatrighttexas.org
Web site: www.eatrighttexas.org

Utah Dietetic Association
Districts: None
Web site: www.eatrightutah.org

Vermont Dietetic Association
Districts: None
Web site: www.eatrightvt.org

Virginia Dietetic Association
Districts: Blue Ridge, Northern, Rich-
mond, Southwest, Tidewater
Web site: www.eatright-va.org

Washington State Dietetic Association
Districts: Greater Seattle, Greater
Spokane, North Sound, Olympia Area,
South Sound, Southwest
Washington, Tricities, Yakima Valley
Web site: www.nutritionusda.org

West Virginia Dietetic Association
Districts: None
Web site: http://eatrightwv.org

Wisconsin Dietetic Association
Districts: Madison, Milwaukee,
Northern
E-mail: WDA@centurytel.net
Web site: www.eatrightwisc.org

Wyoming Dietetic Association
Districts: None
Web site:
www.wyomingdieteticassociation.com

Appendix D

State Licensure Agency Contacts

Note: For links to online information, visit the Commission on Dietetic Registration Web site (www.cdrnet.org/certifications/licensure/agencylist.cfm).

Alabama
Board of Examiners for Dietetic/
Nutrition Practice
400 South Union Street, Suite 445
Montgomery, AL 36104
Phone: 334/242-4505

Alaska
State of Alaska
Department of Community and
Economic Development
Division of Occupational Licensing
PO Box 110806
Juneau, AK 99811-0806
Phone: 907/465-2580

Arkansas
Arkansas Dietetics Licensure Board
PO Box 1016
North Little Rock, AR 72215
Phone: 501/221-0566

Connecticut
Connecticut Department of Public
Health Dietitian-Nutritionist
Certification
410 Capitol Avenue, MS #12 APP
PO Box 340308
Hartford, CT 06134
Phone: 860/509-7603

Delaware
Attn: Board of Dietetics/Nutrition
Cannon Building, Suite 203
861 Silver Lake Boulevard
Dover, DE 19904
Phone: 302/744-4500

District of Columbia
Department of Health Professional
Licensing Administration
Attn: Dietitian and Nutrition
Renewal Processing
717 14th Street NW, Suite 600
Washington, DC 20005
Phone: 877/672-2174

Florida
Department of Health
4042 Bald Cypress Way
BIN-C 01
Tallahassee, FL 32399
Phone: 850/488-0595

Georgia
Board of Examiners of Licensed
Dietitians
237 Coliseum Drive
Macon, GA 31217
Phone: 478/207-2440

Hawaii
Office of Health Care Assurance
601 Kamokila Blvd. Rm 395
Kapolie, Hawaii 96707
Phone: 808/586-4080

Idaho
Board of Medicine
Dietitian Licensure Board
1755 Westgate Drive
PO Box 83720
Boise, Idaho 83720
Phone: 208/327-7000

Illinois
Department of Financial and Professional
Regulation
320 West Washington, 3rd Floor
Springfield, IL 62786
Phone: 217/782-0800

Indiana
Professional Licensing Agency
ATTN: Indiana Dietitian Certification
Board
402 W. Washington Street, Room W072
Indianapolis, IN 46204
Phone: 317/234-2043

Iowa
Iowa State Board of Dietetics
Bureau of Professional Licensure
Lucas State Office Building
321 East 12th Street, 4th Floor
Des Moines, IA 50319-0075
Phone: 515/281-6959

Kansas
Licensing Administrator
Health Occupations Credentialing
Department of Health and
Environment
Curtis State Office Building
1000 SW Jackson, Suite 200
Topeka, KS 66612-1365
Phone: 785/296-1240

Kentucky
Board Administrator
Board of Licensure and Certification for
Dietitians and Nutritionists
PO Box 1360
Frankfort, KY 40602-1360
Phone: 502/564-3296

Louisiana
Louisiana State Board of Examiners in
Dietetics and Nutrition
18550 Highland Road, Suite B
Baton Rouge, LA 70809
225/756-3490

Maine
Board of Licensing of Dietetic Practice
Office of Licensing and Registration
Department of Professional and Financial
Regulation
35 State House Station
Augusta, ME 04333-0035
Phone: 207/624-8603

Maryland
State Board of Dietetic Practice
Department of Health and Mental
Hygiene
4201 Patterson Avenue, 3rd Floor
Baltimore, MD 21215-2299
Phone: 410/764-4733

Massachusetts
Board of Dietitians and Nutritionists
Division of Professional Licensure
239 Causeway Street
Boston, MA 02114
Phone: 617/727-3074

Michigan
Michigan Dietetic Association (MDA)
c/o Susanne Consiglio, RD, Executive
Director
22811 Greater Mack, Suite 105
St. Clair Shores, MI 48080
Phone: 586/774-7447
(Rules are currently in development.)

Minnesota
Board of Dietetics and Nutrition Practice
2829 University Avenue SE, Suite 555
Minneapolis, MN 55414
Phone: 651/201-2764

Mississippi
Mississippi State Department of Health
Professional Licensure
PO Box 1700
Jackson, MS 39215-1700
Phone: 601/364-7360

Missouri
Missouri Division of Professional
Registration
State Committee of Dietitians
3605 Missouri Boulevard
PO Box 1335
Jefferson City, MO 65102-1335
Phone: 573/522-3438

Montana
Department of Labor and Industry
Board of Medical Examiners
PO Box 200513
301 S. Park Avenue, 4th Floor
Helena, MT 59620-0513
Phone: 406/841-2364

Nebraska
Board of Medical Nutrition Therapy
PO Box 94986
Lincoln, NE 68509-4986
Phone: 402/471-2115

New Hampshire
New Hampshire Board of Licensed
Dietitians
Department of Health and Human
Services
129 Pleasant St.
Concord, NH 03301-5127
Phone: 603/271-0853 or 603/271-0277

New Mexico
State of New Mexico Regulation and
Licensing Department
Nutrition and Dietetics Board
PO Box 25101
Santa Fe, NM 87504
Phone: 505/476-4625

New York
State Board for Dietetics and Nutrition
Education Building West Wing
2nd Floor
89 Washington Avenue
Albany, NY 12234
Phone: 518/474-3817 ext. 560

North Carolina
North Carolina Board of Dietetics and
Nutrition
1500 Sunday Drive, Suite 102
Raleigh, NC 27607
Phone: 919/861-5580

North Dakota
North Dakota Board of Dietetic Practice
PO Box 6142
Grand Forks, ND 58206
Phone: 701/838-2785

Ohio
Ohio Board of Dietetics
77 South High Street, 18th Floor
Columbus, OH 43215-6119
Phone: 614/466-3291

Oklahoma
Oklahoma Board of Medical Licensure
and Supervision
PO Box 18256
Oklahoma City, OK 73154-0256
Phone: 405/848-6841

Oregon
Board of Examiners of Licensed
Dietitians
800 NE Oregon Street, #21, Suite 407
Portland, OR 97232-2187
Phone: 971/673-0190

Pennsylvania
Pennsylvania State Board of Nursing
PO Box 2649
Harrisburg, PA 17105-2649
Phone: 717/783-7142

Puerto Rico
Department of Health
Board of Examiners for Nutritionists and
Dietitians
Call Box 10200
Santurce, PR 00908
Phone: 787/725-7904

Rhode Island
Health Professions Regulation
Rhode Island Department of Health
3 Capitol Hill, Room 105
Providence, RI 02908-5097
Phone: 401/222-5888

South Carolina
South Carolina Panel for Dietetics
Synergy Business Park
Kingstree Building
110 Centerview Dr., Suite 306
Columbia, SC 29210

South Dakota
South Dakota Board of Medical and
Osteopathic Examiners
125 South Main Avenue
Sioux Falls, SD 57104
Phone: 605/367-7781

Tennessee
Board of Dietitian/Nutritionist
Examiners
Cordell Hull Building, 1st Floor
425 5th Avenue North
Nashville, TN 37243
Phone: 615/532-5096

Texas
Texas State Board of Examiners of
Dietitians
1100 W. 49th Street
Austin, TX 78756-3183
Phone: 512/834-6601

Utah
Division of Occupational and
Professional Licensing
Utah Dietitian Licensing Board
PO Box 146741
Salt Lake City, UT 84114-6741
Phone: 801/530-6767

Vermont
Office of Professional Regulation
National Life Building, North FL2
Montpelier, VT 05620-3402
Phone: 802/828-1505

Washington

Washington State Department of Health
Health Professions Quality Assurance
Customer Service Center
PO Box 47865
Olympia, WA 98504-7865
Phone: 360/236-4700

West Virginia

West Virginia Board of Licensed of
Dietitians
723 Kanawha Boulevard East
Room 105 Union Building
Charleston, WV 25301
Phone: 304/558-1024 or 800/293-9832

Wisconsin

Department of Regulation and Licensing
Dietitians Affiliated Credentialing Board
1400 East Washington Avenue
PO Box 8935
Madison, WI 53708-8935
Phone: 608/266-2112

Index